Autoimmune
Diseases and Their
Environmental Triggers

ALSO BY ELAINE A. MOORE
WITH LISA MOORE

Graves' Disease: A Practical Guide
(McFarland, 2001)

Autoimmune Diseases and Their Environmental Triggers

by ELAINE A. MOORE

ILLUSTRATIONS BY MARVIN G. MILLER

McFarland & Company, Inc., Publishers

Jefferson, North Carolina, and London

This book is intended as an educational resource and not as a substitute for medical treatment. Patients with autoimmune disease need to be under the care of a qualified physician or an alternative medicine provider. It is important for all patients to consult with their medical advisors before making any changes in their therapeutic regimen.

Library of Congress Cataloguing-in-Publication Data

Moore, Elaine A., 1948–
    Autoimmune diseases and their environmental triggers / by Elaine A. Moore.
        p.   cm.
    Includes bibliographical references and index.
    ISBN 0-7864-1322-0 (softcover : 50# alkaline paper) ∞
    1. Autoimmune diseases—Popular works.   2. Environ-mentally induced diseases—Popular works.   [DNLM:
1. Autoimmune Diseases—etiology.   2. Autoimmune Diseases—therapy.   3. Complementary Therapies.
4. Environmental Pollutants—adverse effects.
WD 305 M821a 2002]   I. Title.

RC600 .M665 2002
616.97'8—dc21   2002003869

British Library cataloguing data are available

Cover illustrations by Marvin G. Miller

Manufactured in the United States of America

McFarland & Company, Inc., Publishers
    Box 611, Jefferson, North Carolina 28640
    www.mcfarlandpub.com

To Rick

Acknowledgments

I'd like to take this opportunity to thank my husband Rick and my children, Brett and Lisa, for their constant encouragement and support. I also owe special thanks to my many friends and relatives who have autoimmune disease, especially Jody, Drew, Julie, Sally and Maria. Their questions inspired me to explore the origins of the many disorders that target the body's own tissues and cells. The basic question posed to me, often stated as "why me?" sparked my interest and helped frame the chapters of this book.

Many thanks also goes to Deb Howe and the board members of Howe Charities in Lexington, Kentucky, for awarding me an environmental writing grant. Their enthusiasm for this project encouraged me more than they can imagine. And special thanks to Virginia Ladd, President of the American Autoimmune Related Diseases Association (AARDA), for the wealth of information she graciously shared.

I'd also like to express my gratitude to the U.S. National Institutes of Health for allowing me to share the findings presented at the 1998 conference, *Linking Environmental Agents to Autoimmune Disease*, jointly sponsored by the Juvenile Diabetes Foundation International, the U.S. Environmental Protection Agency and AARDA. And thanks to the many scientists who brought these findings to light.

Lastly, I'd like to thank my friend and co-worker, Marvin G. Miller, for his clever illustrations, which once again have helped make a complex subject easy to understand.

Contents

List of Illustrations

Introduction

Most people realize that a high cholesterol level and sedentary lifestyle are risk factors for heart disease. But how many people can recite the risk factors for autoimmune disease (AD)? Then again, how many people know what ADs are?

The generic term "autoimmune disease" refers to a number of different disorders that originate in the immune system. The underlying cause of these disorders is an immune system defect that goads the immune system into deviating from its normal protective functions. Led astray by environmental and genetic influences, the immune system spurs an attack against the body's own tissues and cells.

Simply stated, according to current theory, ADs develop in individuals with a certain combination of genes and lifestyle factors who are exposed to certain environmental triggers. These environmental triggers include hormones, stress, infectious agents, vaccines, heavy metals such as mercury and lead, traumatic injury, ultraviolet radiation and a plethora of industrial, medicinal and agricultural chemicals.

A National Institutes of Health publication, *Understanding Autoimmune Diseases*, advises that physicians warn their autoimmune disease patients about environmental triggers. Avoiding these triggers, this bulletin reports, could prevent symptoms from flaring up or progressing. Unfortunately, however, few patients ever hear this warning.

The Role of Environmental Triggers

Patients hearing this warning might wonder how environmental agents can affect the arthralgia (joint pain and stiffness), fatigue, neurological symptoms and muscle pain that rule their lives. After all, ADs

1

seem to have inexplicable lives of their own, with symptoms that myste-
riously change over time. Periods of remission alternate with periods of
variable symptom severity. In some instances, even the predominant symptoms change over time, with blistering rashes miraculously vanishing only
to be replaced by crippling joint pain.

For many years, patients and their doctors saw no logic to this waxing and waning of symptoms. Now scientists know that a variety of environmental factors influence the immune response, thereby affecting both
the symptoms and the disease course. However, in the early stages of
autoimmune disease, symptoms are often insidious. Thus, when symptoms are easiest to treat and the avoidance of environmental triggers most
likely to elicit remissions, patients aren't often sure if they even need to
see a doctor.

Diagnostic Difficulties

Even when doctors are consulted, early, vague AD symptoms are
likely to be ignored. A survey conducted by the American Autoimmune
Related Diseases Association (AARDA) reported that the medical com-
plaints of women, the prime targets of AD, are often dismissed. Many
survey respondents stated that, before their diagnoses, they were regarded
as hypochondriacs. A number of these women report being treated for
anxiety and given antidepressant drugs. A related AARDA publication
reports that for ADs, an accurate diagnosis takes an average of seven years
and five doctors.

The list of ADs is long and includes diseases as common as insulin
dependent diabetes mellitus, myasthenia gravis and rheumatoid arthritis.
The connective tissue diseases, in particular, often stymie even the most
astute diagnosticians. The rheumatologic autoimmune disorder Sjögren's
syndrome (SS) is particularly difficult to diagnose because many of its
symptoms mimic symptoms seen in other diseases including systemic
lupus erythematosus (SLE) and rheumatoid arthritis (RA). Does it really
matter if a patient has SLE or RA alone, RA or SLE with SS, or SS
alone?

Definitely. Some medications used for treatment of SLE or RA or
even the common cold can exacerbate or worsen symptoms in Sjögren's
syndrome. And whether SS occurs alone or accompanies another AD,
coexisting as a secondary disorder, has much to say about a particular disease's progression and severity.

An early accurate diagnosis and a knowledge of what environmental factors to avoid can make a world of difference in how a particular patient will fare. But unfortunately, the causes of AD are not fully understood, and the list of things to avoid is hardly common knowledge.

The Value of Self-Care

With today's cost crunching medical crisis, patients, especially those with autoimmune disease, must become involved in their own healing plans. It's essential for patients to learn the value of self-care, including the avoidance of environmental triggers and toxins and the adjunctive value of holistic healing. According to Hippocrates in *Airs, Waters, and Places*, the basis of health lies in fresh air, pure food and water, the quality of the land, and the conditions of living quarters.

Health, as Hippocrates originally defined it, requires a harmonious integration of environmental and social factors. Hippocrates recognized the healing forces inherent in every living organism, which he called nature's healing power. Of pertinence to ADs, this sage healer elaborated on the body's specific requirement for balance or equilibrium between its "humors" and its "passions." This balance, he explained, is essential for chemical and hormonal balance to exist. And as we'll learn later in this book, these humors, passions and hormones have a profound influence on our immune system health and AD development.

Putting the Links Together

Although there have been tremendous advances in finding the genes associated with ADs (see chapter 4), the research spotlight is currently focused on environmental triggers. In September of 1998, in a conference sponsored by several agencies including the National Institute of Environmental Health Sciences (NIEHS) and AARDA, molecular biologists, immunologists, toxicologists and other researchers gathered in Research Triangle Park, North Carolina, for the purpose of discussing these environmental concerns. Their findings (see chapter 5) form the foundation for the specific environmental autoimmune disease triggers described in this book.

Etiology and Treatment

Etiology refers to the causes of disease. The etiology of ADs includes both genetic and environmental factors. The early chapters of this book explain how environmental agents can disrupt the immune system and induce AD development.

In describing how ADs develop, I open doors to healing options. It's important to understand how environmental agents alter the immune system's cells and chemicals, precipitating and perpetuating the disease process. Armed with this knowledge, patients can understand how important it is to avoid environmental triggers, and how treatment options as diverse as stress reduction techniques and monoclonal antibody can alter the immune response and aid the healing process.

Chapter 6 describes diagnostic criteria as well as the various tests used to aid in diagnosis, while chapter 7 describes the main classifications and subtypes of AD. Chapters 8 and 9 describe traditional allopathic and alternative treatment approaches.

Autoimmune Diseases and Their Environmental Triggers explores the link between ADs and environmental triggers while describing the problems inherent in compiling a comprehensive list of these triggers. While certain chemicals and drugs described in this book are intimately linked to AD development, most chemicals have never been studied for their immune system effects.

The problems in identifying environmental triggers are discussed, along with current research trends, in chapter 10, followed by a chapter listing resources, including publications, support groups, references, internet web sites and support groups.

1

Health vs. Environment

The term "autoimmune disease" (AD) refers to a number of unrelated disorders with one common link. They're all caused by an immune system defect that causes the body to attack its own tissues. The list of ADs includes conditions as diverse as type 1 or insulin dependent diabetes mellitus (IDDM), multiple sclerosis (MS), and Peyronie's disease, a rare disorder affecting the connective tissue supporting the penis.

Approximately twenty percent of the population is susceptible to developing ADs. That is, these individuals possess certain genes that predispose them to developing autoimmune diseases. However, only 3 percent to 5 percent of the population goes on to develop autoimmune disorders.

According to current theory, individuals who develop AD do so because they're exposed to certain environmental triggers. Residents of the U.S. and Europe have a far greater likelihood of developing ADs than individuals residing in Third World countries. The progress of the industrial revolution, it seems, has more than one consequence.

CELLS AND SAND

Imagine relaxing on a sandy beach building a sandcastle. You border the moat with seashells and frame the windows with pebbles. Alas, the wind picks up. Pale granules shimmy away in a cloud of dust. Suddenly, the sky darkens and rain begins to pour. Grains of sand become toffee colored sand pearls. The castle sags. By the time you've rolled up your blanket and batted off the sand, your castle is a lump of mud.

Although the human body doesn't crumble when it rains, in many ways it's similar to our imaginary castle. Sandcastles are formed by a collection of dampened sand granules surrounded by and linked to moats.

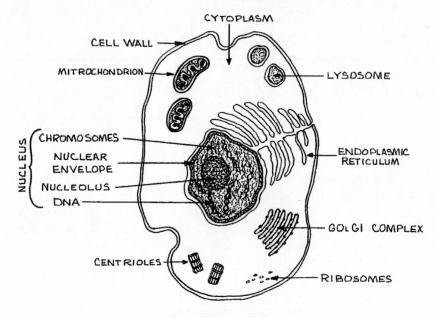

Basic Human Cell

The body is composed of cells, clustered into tissues and organs linked together by the circulatory and lymphatic systems.

Each granule of sand affects the castle's overall structure, and each cell contributes to the body's overall structure and function. When the castle's steeples collapse, the drawbridge caves in. Cellular changes affecting one organ, for instance the thyroid or the pancreas, eventually affect all other bodily systems. Shifting sand may initially go unnoticed. And the body's cellular changes, especially those induced by the immune system, may not be detected until the consequences are akin to a squashed castle.

WHAT IS THE IMMUNE SYSTEM?

The immune system, described further in chapter 3, refers to an intricately related army of organs, cells, and chemical molecules scattered throughout the body. All of the immune system components work in conjunction to protect the body from foreign substances, particularly viruses and bacteria, and to inhibit cellular changes that ultimately lead to the development of tumors or autoimmunity.

All of the body's tissues, including blood, are made up of small specialized structures known as cells. The immune system's key players are cells known as white blood cells or leukocytes. Although leukocytes originate in the bone marrow, they eventually travel to the blood, where they freely circulate. They also travel to various immune system organs, such as lymph nodes, where they're stored until needed.

What Does the Immune System Do Anyway?

The immune system has two primary functions or job descriptions, which immune system cells perform in a series of steps known as an immune response.

(1) Immune system cells, particularly leukocytes known as macrophages, protect us from foreign substances (protein, carbohydrate or lipid particles, for instance, protein particles present in bacteria and viruses) by rushing to the point of attack, barring entry and causing inflammation. If this strategy proves ineffective, other leukocytes, particularly helper T lymphocyte cells, rush forward, initiating their defense by multiplying, releasing potent chemicals, and forming protective proteins known as antibodies. Antibodies offer protection because they're capable of attacking and destroying these foreign substances the next time they come around.

(2) Immune system cells with suppressor or cytotoxic functions (capable of destroying other cells) stop the growth of neoplastic or cancerous tissue cells, preventing tumor development. They also destroy any infected cells, and they normally prevent other immune system cells from becoming autoreactive and producing antibodies directed toward one's own body (autoantibodies). Thus, a healthy immune system prevents infections, tumor growth, and autoimmune disease development.

What Is Immunity?

If we're immune to something or someone, for instance an old love, their presence has no effect on us. We might notice them, but we don't respond. If the wind had no effect on our sandcastle, we would say that our castle is immune to the wind. If we develop chicken pox, our immune system produces antibodies to the Varicella zoster virus, the infective agent in chicken pox. These specific Varicella antibodies provide immunity, protecting us from contracting chicken pox.

In other words, our having previously had chicken pox makes us immune from developing it a second time since we developed antibodies to chicken pox when we were initially infected. If we're exposed to chicken pox again, our immune system cells, which have the capability of memory, recognize these Varicella viruses. Consequently, our immune cells produce even more Varicella zoster antibodies.

When we're vaccinated against a specific disease, we receive minute amounts of the infectious agent. For instance in the chicken pox vaccine, we're inoculated with tiny amounts of live Varicella virus. The live virus in vaccines is inactivated and suspended in a solution of various chemicals, including mercury, formaldehyde and tin. When we're vaccinated, our immune systems recognize the infectious material in the vaccine as a foreign antigen attacking us. In response, our immune system cells produce antibodies.

Antibody Titers

A subsequent vaccine known as a booster shot causes our immune system to step up antibody production. Our immune system recognizes booster shots as a subsequent invasion. The more antibodies we have, the higher our antibody titer. This means that laboratory technicians can detect these antibodies even when the blood sample is diluted. The highest dilution in which antibodies are still detected is known as the titer. High antibody titers confer better or stronger immunity. If we have high titers of Varicella antibodies and are later exposed to chicken pox, our antibodies destroy any viruses that happen to enter our body. This provides immunity against our developing chicken pox.

However, as adults, especially adults with ADs, we may later develop shingles, a condition also caused by the Varicella virus. Furthermore, adults exposed to children recently vaccinated against Varicella sometimes develop shingles.

Antigens

Any molecule capable of causing an immune system response is known as an antigen. Even tiny tissue particles can act as antigens. Food can also be antigenic, triggering an immune response, unless it's digested and broken down into its amino acid building blocks before reaching the

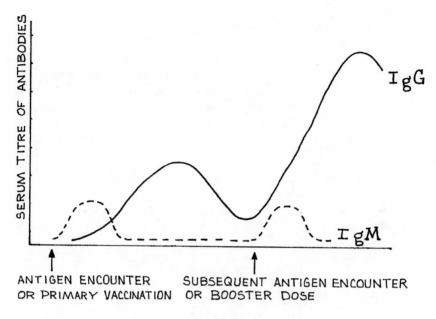

Antibody Titres

circulation. With millions of different antigens to watch out for, how does the immune system distinguish between our body's own antigens and antigens that are foreign threats?

Self-Tolerance

The answer lies in marker molecules. Each specific antigen has distinct molecules or markers on its surface that the immune system recognizes. All of our body's cellular or tissue antigens have the same specific markers, which the immune system recognizes as "self" markers. Our immune systems have self-tolerance, meaning that our immune system tolerates or ignores self-antigens. Viral and bacterial cells have their own distinct markers, which the immune system recognizes as "non-self" or foreign. The immune system does not tolerate these foreign antigens.

WHEN THE IMMUNE SYSTEM FAILS US

Normally, the immune system organs and cells work together to keep us healthy. Disorders occur when the immune system is hyperactive and overreacts and also when the immune system is suppressed or underactive, and thereby ineffective.

• When the immune system underreacts or fails to recognize external foreign antigens, such as viruses, infection results.
• If the immune system fails to react to an abnormal internal antigen, for instance an abnormal cell growth, the result is cancer.
• If the immune system overreacts to an external antigen such as pollen, allergy results.
• And when certain helper type immune system cells mistakenly overreact to one's own tissue cells, or when other protective immune system cells become weakened or diminished in number and fail to destroy autoreactive cells (cells activated to react against self components), the result is autoimmune disease.

Consequences and Symptoms

When immune system cells react inappropriately in any of the ways described above, the initial symptoms are often vague. By the time symptoms become overt or pronounced, cellular damage may be considerable. For instance, in acquired immune deficiency syndrome (AIDS) and in malignant cancers, symptoms may go unnoticed until the disease progresses to an advanced stage. Although ADs aren't the same as cancer or AIDS, the underlying defect in all of these disorders is immune system dysfunction.

In ADs, common symptoms such as muscle weakness or rash often emerge so subtly they're never suspected of being even remotely linked to disease. Adding to their innocuousness, symptoms in the early stages of AD seldom show signs of progressive worsening. In fact, variable periods of severity and remission and changes in predominant symptoms over time are autoimmune hallmarks. It's hardly surprising that autoimmune diseases are difficult to diagnose. Consider my story.

A GENETIC LEGACY

An extremely light-sensitive child, I squinted so fiercely I developed a forehead furrow before second grade. Teachers and bus drivers frequently asked me what was wrong. Often, they remarked that I looked as if I were about to cry. Since I was generally happy or at least not unhappy, I learned to avert my gaze or bury my head in a book.

Compounding my light sensitivity or photophobia, I had a staring problem. My normal expression, vacuous and wide-eyed, made me look startled. Years later, I learned that this stare often accompanies autoimmune thyroid disease (AITD). Despite these and many other symptoms, I was nearly forty before I was diagnosed with Graves' disease (GD), an autoimmune hyperthyroid disorder that may also affect the muscles and eyes.

Risk Factors

Often, especially in a migratory population accustomed to consulting various specialists, it can be difficult to link all the pieces of one's medical history. After all, it's not unusual for patients to simultaneously consult different doctors for different ailments. When their ADs are finally diagnosed, they realize that all their separate ailments were actually early symptoms of their particular autoimmune disease.

My risk factors for AITD, or diagnostic clues, included family history of autoimmune disease, lifelong allergies and anaphylactic reactions, target age and sex, prematurely graying hair (typically seen in AITD), and numerous environmental triggers, including significant chemical exposure.

In the Great Lakes region where I grew up, I regularly ate fish that were likely chemically contaminated (see chapter 5), and my neighborhood was regularly blasted with pesticides. And for more than 20 years I worked as a chemist, using a variety of toxic chemicals and organic solvents since found to cause immune system harm.

My co-worker Jill, diagnosed at 20 with Addison's disease, an AD causing adrenal insufficiency, reported that since childhood people often complimented her bronze skin coloring, commenting that it set off her blue eyes. Only later did she learn that her skin tone was an early hint of Addison's disease. Before her diagnosis, she was treated for a litany of ailments that turned out to be symptoms of adrenal insufficiency.

When Jill later developed Hashimoto's thyroiditis, she discovered it inadvertently by running her own thyroid function tests at work. For several years, Jill had complained of symptoms of hypothyroidism, symptoms her doctor blamed on her Addison's disease.

INCIDENCE

Some patients, especially those with long-term chronic ADs like type 1 diabetes (also known as juvenile or insulin dependent diabetes mellitus or IDDM) or pernicious anemia (PA), may not even realize that they have an AD since the autoimmune nature of these disorders has only recently been discovered.

An Autoimmune Epidemic in the Western World

In 1970, when I was studying laboratory medicine, ADs were confined to a handful of what were then called collagen disorders. Although other ADs such as IDDM existed, the autoimmune nature of these disorders was not yet recognized. IDDM was considered a disorder of deficient insulin secretion. However, no one knew that antibodies that destroyed the insulin secreting cells of the pancreas were responsible.

In 1970, the clinical laboratory only offered about 10 different diagnostic autoantibody tests that were routinely sent out to the country's major reference laboratories. Furthermore, doctors rarely ordered these tests and results were seldom positive. In-house, we occasionally performed lupus erythematosus (LE) prep tests to help diagnose systemic lupus erythematosus (SLE). We rarely saw positive preps.

In 1998, Dr. Noel Rose, a Professor of Immunology at Johns Hopkins University and consultant for the American Autoimmune Related Disease Association (AARDA), reported that more than 10 million Americans suffer from the major ADs, such as multiple sclerosis (MS). Dr. Rose defines ADs as diseases that have animal models in which disease can be induced in animals under similar conditions. AARDA founder Virginia Ladd reports that when you consider all ADs, including those, such as fibromyalgia and chronic fatigue disease, for which animal models have not yet been demonstrated, the number of Americans with ADs rises to upwards of 50 million.

ADs are primarily seen in the Western world. Of interest, immigrants take on the same incidence of the disease as the native or indigenous population, often exceeding it. Whether the differences in AD incidence between Western and Third World nations are due to sociological, nutritional, parasitic or hygienic reasons remains unclear. The primary candidates, however, are viruses, bacteria, and other environmental factors.

ENVIRONMENTAL TRIGGERS

If you happen to be struck by a car, there's no question about what caused your medical maladies. However, if you develop an AD it's nearly impossible to pinpoint a specific cause. Finding the specific environmental trigger is for the most part impossible, especially considering the many years it often takes for ADs to be correctly diagnosed.

How do we know that environmental factors are involved in AD development? A number of specific environmental triggers have been studied and found to contribute to certain specific ADs. For instance, silica is known to trigger scleroderma.

Many other substances are strongly suspected of causing AD and of exacerbating symptoms. Sunlight exacerbates symptoms in system lupus erythematosus and ultraviolet light and heat are associated with exacerbating MS symptoms. Vaccines to diphtheria, tetanus and polio are known to trigger Guillain-Barré syndrome, and the rubella virus along with several vaccines are thought by some researchers to trigger the development of IDDM (see chapter 5).

Drug Related Autoimmune Disease

A diverse group of environmental compounds, including many common prescription medications, can trigger AD development. For instance, the heart medication procainamide can cause lupus-like symptoms, including arthralgia and joint pain. Although symptoms of drug related lupus generally resolve when the offending drug is withdrawn, immune system changes may persist (also see chapter 5).

Also, some drugs and microorganisms complex with the body's own protein particles or self-antigens. For instance, in autoimmune hemolytic anemia (AIHA), certain drugs alter the surface of erythrocytes (red blood cells or RBCs). Normally, RBCs have surface markers such as blood type and Rh factor. Altered by drugs, the RBC cell provides a new carrier for an Rh antigen hapten that stimulates the immune system to produce RBC autoantibodies. The antihypertensive (blood pressure lowering) agent alpha-methyldopa is most often implicated, although other drugs, including antibiotics and quinines, are associated with the development of AIHA.[1]

The Importance of Recognizing Environmental Triggers

Most people realize that asbestos causes respiratory diseases and lung cancer, and that lead toxicity cripples mental development. Government regulations have reduced their presence in the environment. Consequently, the number of asbestos and lead associated disorders has significantly declined. Awareness and avoidance of environmental AD triggers has a similar effect.

In 1989, tryptophan, an amino acid and popular health food supplement, was found to cause an AD known as eosinophilic myalgia or myositis that targets white blood cells known as eosinophils. Initially only certain sources of tryptophan were thought to be contaminated, but this hasn't been confirmed. It's currently suspected that tryptophan itself is an AD trigger. Consequently, tryptophan is no longer sold as a health food supplement in the United States and the incidence of eosinophilic myalgia has declined.

The heaviest concentrations of Great Lakes contaminants occurred between 1950 and 1970. In response, government officials ordered a chemical overhaul of the area and a 1976 ban in the U.S. on the use of polychlorinated biphenyls (PCBs), chemicals that are known to interfere with endocrine function. Studies conducted in the last two decades indicate that, although many of these contaminants still persist because they degrade slowly, their concentrations have been dramatically reduced. As a consequence, bird and animal populations native to the Great Lakes region are showing signs of recovery.

Nevertheless, a 1998 Cornell University publication reports that environmental pollution and the degradation of toxic chemicals still cause 40 percent of deaths worldwide. This report, which offers an analysis of population trends, climate change, increasing population and emerging diseases, reports that disease prevalence is worsened by the unprecedented increase in air, water and soil pollutants.[2]

CALL IT PROGRESS

In the years following World War II, Americans fell heir to an assortment of new pesticides, cleaning agents, fertilizers, vaccines and a wide array of turbo-charged industrial chemicals. Medicine cabinets bulged with potent new medicines and freezers became laden with pre-packaged chemically preserved processed foods. However, this chemical cascade has had a price. In this same time frame, particularly in the last two decades of the 20th century, Americans have also witnessed an unprecedented, inexplicably dramatic rise in the incidence of autoimmune disease.

The Vaccine Controversy

The incidence of IDMM rose 6-fold between 1958 and 1998. According to recent studies, some autistic disorders also show evidence of autoimmunity. And the California Education Department reports nearly a 4-fold increase in the number of California children with autistic disorders in the period between April 1993 and April 1998.[3]

Reports of medical experts and emotional testimony from parents of autistic children presented at congressional hearings in the summer of 2000 suggest that certain vaccines may be responsible. Congressman Dan Burton, whose grandson developed autism shortly after receiving a vaccine, stated that he blames the vaccine. Congressman Burton also criticized the fact that members of Atlanta's Centers for Disease Control's (CDC) investigative group, which initially disputed the vaccine-autism link, had financial ties to the vaccine industry at the time their report was presented.

Dr. Andrew J. Wakefield of the Royal Free and University College Medical School in London also testified at the congressional hearing. He identified a link between vaccines and a syndrome of autistic enterocolitis, a gastrointestinal disorder that he was the first to describe. In 1998 he presented a report of 12 affected patients in the prestigious medical journal *Lancet*.[4] He believes his studies pinpoint the vaccine as an environmental trigger for autism.[5]

In a meeting held on 23 October 2000 at the National Institute of Environmental Health Sciences (NIEHS), exchanges between parents/advocates and researchers offered insight into the needs of the people affected by autism. Representatives from the NIEHS and several advocacy groups met to discuss ways to increase research efforts, improve clinical testing, and reduce or eliminate the environmental toxic exposures that may cause or aggravate neurological developmental conditions.

At this conference, Sallie Bernard, executive director of Sensible Action For Ending Mercury-Induced Neurological Disorders, a parent group advocating for the elimination of mercury from vaccines said, "The appearance of signs of autism occurs in a significant number of children who develop and behave normally until being immunized."[6] The CDC is currently evaluating the safety of ethylmercury, a component of thimerosal, which is used as a preservative in vaccines and is suspected of triggering autism.

Autoimmune Disease in Children

The dramatic rise in AD in the last two decades can be partially attributed to an increased life span. The elderly, whose numbers have grown, are indeed more susceptible to developing ADs. With age, the powers of the immune system begin to fail. Protective mechanisms that normally prevent AD become ineffective. However, there is also a disturbing increase in the number of children being diagnosed with ADs.

Today, many children are being diagnosed with juvenile arthritis, SLE, and Graves' disease (GD). Two decades ago, GD in children was considered extremely rare. In the last few years, one small Italian village reported three cases of GD in children less than 3 years old.[7]

2

What Are Autoimmune Diseases?

What are the immunological ramifications of kissing a toad? Kiss a toad and your immune system cells might not tell, but like seasoned voyeurs, the ever-vigilant immune system cells know every detail. As members of the immune system army, the epithelial, macrophage and dendritic cells that form the outer layers of your skin, including your lips, act as border patrol soldiers, barring entry of anything considered "non-self."

Every tissue cell in your body has the same genetic material in its cell nucleus, and this material is distinctly different from anyone else's. The body's white blood cells also have identical genetic markers on their outer surface. Your immune cells are privy to this information. They recognize these genetic markers and, subsequently, regard the toad's or, for that matter, anyone else's cells as foreign, that is, "non-self."

HORROR AUTOTOXICUS

Early in the 1900s, the renowned German physician and scientist Paul Ehrlich (1854-1915) recognized that the amazing ability of the immune system to differentiate "self" from foreign or "non-self" molecules made an attack against the body's own tissues not only possible but inevitable. Realizing the devastation such an attack could cause, Ehrlich coined the term "horror autotoxicus."[1] Until well into the early 1970s, this term was used to describe disorders suspected of having an autoimmune origin.

Discrimination in the Immune System

The immune system has powers of selective discrimination. In other words, immune system cells are able to distinguish one's own cells and tissues from foreign protein molecules. Immune system cells (described further in the next chapter) spend their days scouting for and protecting us from foreign antigens.

Antigenic Determinants

Antigens have markers on their surface known as epitopes or antigenic determinants. These are the specific parts of the antigen that the immune system recognizes and distinguishes as self or foreign.

Some immune system cells, particularly the scavenger white blood cells known as macrophages, don't watch for specific foreign antigens. These cells exert a generalized attack against any antigen they perceive as foreign. Macrophages also scout for virally or bacterially infected cells, which they are able to engulf and destroy. The T lymphocyte white blood cells, however, are programmed to look for specific antigens.

With thousands of different antigens to watch out for, our immune system cells occasionally err. Sometimes, they confuse the protein present in our tissues and cells with foreign antigens. When the immune system attacks self-antigens, the end result is AD. This chapter focuses on the characteristic immune system changes, symptoms and natural course of ADs as well as their incidence and prevalence.

THE BODY'S DEFENSE SYSTEM

As mentioned, our skin's epithelial cells bar external antigens from bodily entry. In addition, white blood cells, especially lymphocytes, travel freely through the circulation and patrol the body's inner sanctions.

Although some cells aggregate or gather at strategic ambush points in lymph nodes or in discrete cellular patches located in our stomach lining, tonsils, adenoids and spleen, most immune system cells keep on the move. White blood cells circulate through the blood, making a clean sweep through the body every 30 minutes. These cells respond to foreign antigens that gain entry via injections, wounds, and transfusions. They

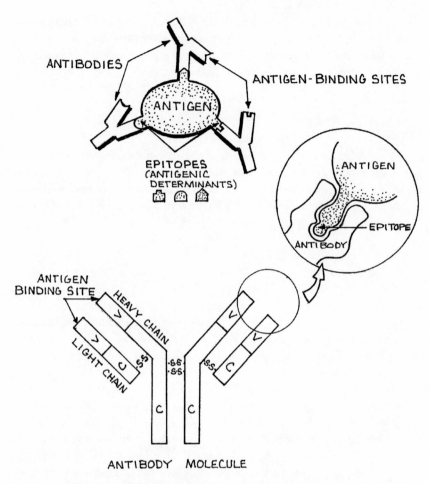

Antigen-Antibody Reaction and Immunoglobulin Structure

also recognize and destroy other white blood cells that have been infected by foreign antigens.

The Non-Specific or Generalized Attack

Upon initiating a generalized attack, tissue cells, particularly macrophages, rush to the site of invasion. For instance, when we're bitten by a bug, these immune cells rush to the skin and dermal layers of the puncture wound and cause inflammation.

The inflammatory response is an effective weapon. It stomps out foreign organisms early in an invasion, confining them to a localized area. However, some stealthy foreign antigens may survive this attack. Furthermore, some of these sequestered foreign antigens may initiate immune changes that promote autoimmune disease.

The Specific Attack

When foreign antigens survive the non-specific attack, the immune system's cellular troops come out in full force. In a separate subsequent reaction, T lymphocytes initiate their own immune response, multiplying to increase their forces. T lymphocytes also initiate a series of events that result in antibody production.

Invisible Defenders

Adept at spying in our defense, our body's immune system cells react to everything that we're exposed to. Besides the epithelial cells, which offer protection through the skin, and the white blood cells, which circulate through the blood or aggregate in tissue, the cells lining the respiratory system also provide a barrier.

Although we generally take it for granted, the respiratory system traps foreign antigens through our nasal hairs and produces mucus, which further blocks foreign antigen entry. The cilia, tiny hair-like projections lining the respiratory tract, filter out foreign particles, initiating a reaction that causes expulsion of the foreign substance through coughing or sneezing.

Like the grains of sand in our imaginary castle, our body's immune system cells react to everything we experience. We might not notice or remember the invisible airborne particles we inhale as we breathe or the anxiety we feel when we're rushed, but the immune system is affected. Just how the immune system is affected can be gauged by measuring levels of white blood cells in the circulation before and after these events and observing changes in the amounts and types of chemical molecules they release.

Gastrointestinal Tract Cells

In their effort to protect us from toxins, our immune system cells also react to every molecule of food, drug or liquid that we ingest. Immune system cells line the gastrointestinal (GI) tract, clustering in discrete patches. Upon recognizing toxins, these cells produce strong stomach acids to destroy them, or they expel the toxins by inducing vomiting. In response to intolerant molecules, the gastric parietal cells can initiate autoantibody production or inflammation.

For instance, individuals who have gluten sensitivity enteropathy (GSE or celiac disease) react to gluten, the protein component of wheat, rye, barley and oats. In response, immune system cells in their intestines produce gliadin, endoymysial, and reticulin autoantibodies. These autoantibodies react against cells in the intestines, destroying the stomach villi and causing nutrient malabsorption.

The body's tissue and organ cells also respond to the cells present in transplant organs or blood transfusions. The same genes that control the immune system (see chapter 4) determine tissue compatibility, or tissue rejection.

IMMUNE PROTECTION AND CONFUSION

Remember how the immune system cells rushed to investigate the toad kiss we encountered at the beginning of the chapter? Normally, immune cells don't miss a trick. The smallest particle of pollen can't slip past without their noticing. Millions of different immune system cells are on constant surveillance.

Considering the abundance of environmental antigens present in our food, water, and even the air we breathe, how can our immune system cells possibly react to all the foreign substances we encounter? The answer is that they can't. Our immune system genes determine what protein particles we'll react to and also how severely we'll react to a particular substance. Furthermore, our genetic makeup helps determine which particular autoimmune diseases we're likely to develop.

Immune System Activity

In ADs, immune system cells overreact to substances they might ordinarily tolerate. For example, in a hyperactive response to that friendly toad, the body's immune cells would produce toad antibodies targeting any toads brave enough to come around again. And in their frenzy to produce antibodies, these hyper cells might also produce autoantibodies against the lips kissed by the toad.

Autoreactive Cells

When the immune system's T lymphocyte cells become confused or tricked, they have the potential to react against "self" components or antigens. These "autoreactive" T cells eventually initiate a chain of events that leads to autoantibody production.

Environmental triggers can cause T cells to become autoreactive. Viruses and bacterial antigens are some of the best known triggers. Have you ever noticed how spiders and ants try to scurry away as you try to eradicate them? Viruses and bacteria have the same instinct for self-preservation. However, these microorganisms are apparently smarter. Bacteria and viruses go to great lengths to survive, especially in their favorite hosts, the human body. One of their favorite tricks is to alter their own DNA.

Molecular Mimicry

On occasion, invasive viruses or bacteria induce changes or mutations in some of the body's own protein molecules or antigens. These altered self-antigens are recognized as foreign. Infectious agents may also produce and release antigens capable of cross-reacting with the body's self-antigens in a condition known as molecular mimicry. Any of these events can trigger T lymphocyte cells to become autoreactive.

Immunologic Tolerance

Each of the body's cell lines has a certain life span or programmed cell death known as apoptosis. Normally, the immune system destroys or neutralizes autoreactive T cells before their time is up, altering apoptosis in an effort to prevent autoantibody production. The immune system accomplishes this by a number of mechanisms, the most well known being clonal deletion, clonal anergy, and peripheral suppression.

Clonal Deletion

Cells replicate by forming clones. Clonal deletion refers to the destruction of T and B lymphocytes during their maturation. T lymphocytes that bear receptors for self-antigens are normally deleted in the thymus while T cells are undergoing maturation. Studies with mice indicate that autoreactive B cells are deleted in a similar process during their maturation in the bone marrow.

However, there are always a few hardy autoreactive cells that manage to slip through. This is evidenced by the presence of B cells occasionally found in the normal peripheral blood circulation that bear receptors for a variety of self-antigens, including thyroglobulin, collagen, DNA, and myelin. These receptors indicate that the immune system's B lymphocytes have responded to these substances.

Clonal Anergy

Cells may be also inactivated, rather than destroyed. Clonal anergy refers to prolonged or irreversible inactivation of self-reactive lymphocytes. Clonal anergy is induced either during maturation or during encounters with other antigens during the process of second signaling, a secondary process required for autoantibody production. According to current theory, if B cells encounter antigen before they are fully mature, an antigen presenting complex (APC) is formed, but the immunoglobulin receptors needed for autoantibody production are never expressed.

Cell Destruction

Autoreactive cells that manage to survive can also be suppressed or destroyed by cytotoxic T lymphocytes (CTLs) and the chemicals, such as cytokines, that they secrete. The loss of immunologic tolerance caused by a failure in any of these mechanisms leads to the production of autoreactive cells, which ultimately leads to autoantibody formation.

ANTIBODIES AND AUTOANTIBODIES

Antibodies are protein molecules produced by immune system cells. Antibodies are made from a type of protein known as immunoglobulin (Ig). Thus, antibodies are also referred to as immunoglobulins. The body normally has a certain amount of immunoglobulin protein. If immunoglobulin levels are low, the body can't fight infection and it becomes susceptible to disease.

Immunoglobulin proteins consist of connected amino acids linked together to form two heavy and two light chains. Five different classes of immunoglobulins exist, depending on the specific amino acids that join

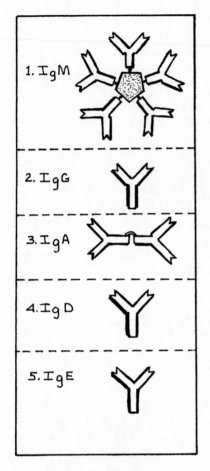

1. I$_g$M

2. I$_g$G

3. I$_g$A

4. I$_g$D

5. I$_g$E

Immunoglobulin classes

together to form the protein molecules in the heavy chains: immunoglobulin G (IgG), M (IgM), E (IgE), A (IgA), and D (IgD). Each of the immunoglobulin classes has their own specific functions. Immunoglobulins produced in response to an allergic reaction belong to the E class (IgE antibodies).

IgG antibodies

Most autoantibodies are IgG immunoglobulins. IgG immunoglobulins are the only immunoglobulins that can cross the placental membrane. Thus, mothers are able to transfer antibodies, including autoantibodies, to their offspring. IgG antibodies confer transient immune protection (or transient disease symptoms). With a half-life (time when total amount is reduced by half) of only 23 days, IgG immunoglobulins only last for about 120 days before their protein molecules begin to break down.

When autoreactive T lymphocytes are tolerated, they initiate a cascade of events that culminates in autoantibody production. Dr. Noel Rose reports that almost everyone has some naturally occurring autoantibodies. When individuals have autoantibodies, but no symptoms of autoimmune disease, they are said to have autoimmunity.

Autoimmunity

Autoimmunity isn't a disease. Nor is it a disorder. It's a benign state in which autoantibodies happen to be present in the circulation. Although most individuals aren't tested for autoantibodies unless they have symptoms of disease, many normal individuals have autoantibodies. These individuals have autoimmunity but not autoimmune disease.

However, when autoantibodies cause symptoms associated with their presence, the patient is said to have an autoimmune disease. Hundreds of different autoantibodies exist, and most, but not all of them, are known to cause specific symptoms. Most patients with autoimmune disease have several different kinds of autoantibodies.

Low titers of thyroglobulin antibodies are found in 30 percent of normal elderly women. These women are said to have evidence of thyroid autoimmunity, but they do not have autoimmune thyroid disease.

Autoimmune Diseases

Symptoms in the various ADs often overlap. Similar to what is seen in non-autoimmune diseases, certain symptoms, such as headache, may occur in several different autoimmune disorders. Despite the diagnostic confusion caused by this overlap, each AD has its own characteristic chemical and immunological profiles and its own cluster of symptoms. However, considerable variation may be seen among patients. For instance, not all patients with systemic lupus erythematosus have kidney involvement.

Cell Receptors and Autoantibodies

Hormones and medications cause specific, not random or haphazard, effects. In order for chemical molecules to activate cells, causing biological actions such as pain relief, chemicals must react with specific receptors located on various cells.

Receptors refer to the specific cell component, usually a protein that hormones and other chemicals bind with. Cell receptors may be introverts hiding inside the cell's nucleus or they may be extroverts clinging to the cell's surface. For instance, thyroid hormone causes effects by binding and activating specific thyroid hormone receptors located on tissue cells throughout the body. Thyroid hormone causes a rise in heart rate when it activates thyroid hormone receptors present in the heart.

Autoantibodies can interfere with the effects of hormones by mimicking hormones and binding to cell receptors in place of the intended substance. For instance, certain thyroid autoantibodies can block thyroid hormone, causing symptoms of hormone deficiency. Autoantibodies can also destroy receptors, interfering with biological actions. An example is myasthenia gravis, where autoantibodies destroy acetylcholine receptors, interfering with the normal transmission of neuromuscular impulses.

HOW SYMPTOMS DEVELOP

Symptoms in AD can be caused by white blood cells infiltrating tissue and causing inflammation or by autoantibodies blocking or reacting with cell receptors. Also, during an immune response, immune system cells can release chemicals, such as complement or cytokines, that destroy tissue components or other cells.

Immune Complexes

Autoantibodies can also form lattice-like immune complexes with antigens or complement. Immune complexes can lodge between tissue cells preventing normal cell function. Generally a poor prognostic sign when they circulate through the body as a complex, autoantibodies are particularly destructive, especially to the kidneys.

Occasionally, symptoms result from the combined efforts of autoantibodies and immune system chemicals. In autoimmune hemolytic anemia, for example, red blood cells are destroyed by antibody-induced, complement-mediated lysis (rupture or destruction of the intact cell). In this case, antibody and complement work together.

IMMUNE MECHANISMS IN AUTOIMMUNE DISEASE

Autoimmune disease results from three different immune mechanisms:

(1) antibody-mediated cytotoxicity, in which antibodies are directed against cell surface self-antigens; examples include myasthenia gravis and Graves' disease.
(2) cell-mediated hypersensitivities, such as IDDM and MS, which are mediated by a type of lymphocyte known as CD4 T helper cells. These responses are also known as delayed hypersensitivities because it takes several days for the immune response, often virally-induced, to produce autoantibodies.

(3) Immune complex disorders where damage is caused when antigen-antibody complexes lodge in tissue; an example is the kidney or renal disease associated with SLE.

Humoral Immunity

When autoantibodies are responsible for symptoms, the cause is humoral-mediated immunity, which is an adapted or acquired response. In humoral immunity, programmed T cells with the capability of memory are taught to target specific antigens, producing antibodies or autoantibodies if the system is flawed.

Autoantibodies may target certain organs or they may be associated with a particular disease, although their function is sometimes unclear. For instance, antimitochondrial antibodies (AMA) are seen in nearly all cases of primary biliary cirrhosis (PBC) although their function is unknown.

Cellular or Native Immunity

When macrophages engulf and destroy tissue cells and induce the production and release of other cytotoxic (capable of destroying cells) lymphocytes (CTLs), the resulting AD is said to be caused by cell-mediated immunity.

Some ADs, such as SLE, are caused by a combination of humoral and cell mediated immunity. Immune complexes that lodge in tissue and induce damage via activation of complement molecules and white blood cell infiltration can also cause symptoms in SLE and other disorders. The disease process in SLE, however, is initiated primarily by antibodies and is not considered a classic T cell disease.

SYSTEMIC VS. ORGAN SPECIFIC DISEASES

ADs may be classified into two major types, *systemic* and *organ specific*. In systemic diseases, the immune system targets the cells of several different specific organs. An example is SLE in which cells of the lungs, skin, joints and kidneys may be affected. In organ specific diseases, one specific organ is generally targeted. For instance, in the autoimmune thyroid diseases (AITDs), the immune system targets the thyroid gland, causing either hypothyroidism or hyperthyroidism.

Most organ specific diseases target the endocrine glands, although any of the body's organs may be affected. For instance, myositis targets muscles and pemphigoid diseases affect the skin. In some disorders, such as hypoparathyroidism or multiple sclerosis, there may be variable etiologies or causes. In some cases the disorder has an autoimmune origin and in others, there is no immune system involvement.

CLASSIFICATION OF AUTOIMMUNE DISEASES

Autoimmune diseases have traditionally been classified according to the major organ systems that they affect. The primary classifications include connective tissue, nervous system components, endocrine glands, the skin, mucous membranes, the liver, the gastrointestinal system, blood vessels, the eyes, the genital system, and the brain, although any of the body's tissues and cells may be affected. See also chapter 7.

Primary Diseases and Associated Syndromes

Some ADs may occur as either primary diseases or as a syndrome accompanying other ADs. For instance, Sjögren's syndrome, which primarily affects the oral and ocular glands, occurs in many patients with autoimmune thyroid disease or rheumatoid arthritis. Sjögren's syndrome can also occur as a primary connective tissue disease in which auditory, gastric and vaginal glands may also be affected.

NATURAL COURSE AND STAGES OF AUTOIMMUNE DISEASE

AD symptoms have a tendency to wax and wane. In other words, symptoms don't necessarily progressively worsen, although they may. Usually, symptoms tend to fluctuate, increasing in times of stress and exposure to other environmental triggers. Most ADs are associated with a cluster of symptoms that appear sporadically, allowing the patient variable periods of severity and remission. Occasionally, only one predominant symptom may occur, although symptoms may change over time, confusing diagnosis.

In some systemic diseases, such as SLE, disease severity and progression depend on which organ system is primarily targeted. Most of the morbidity and mortality of SLE are seen in patients who develop renal disease, even though new renal treatment regimens have greatly improved disease outcome.

Not all ADs are unpredictable. Some diseases are known to progress in discrete stages. For instance, primary biliary cirrhosis (PBC) has four separate progressive stages, although many patients remain in the early stages for many years with no evidence of disease progression. And patients with AITD frequently have both conditions of autoimmune hypothyroidism and hyperthyroidism at different times in their lifetime depending on the predominant type of thyroid autoantibodies present in the blood.

DEMOGRAPHIC DIFFERENCES

Female Bias

Females of every mammalian species studied demonstrate stronger immune systems than men when challenged with antigens. Females outperform males in tests of immune strength throughout their lifetimes, but especially after puberty. Although the reasons are unclear, estrogen is a likely factor since it's linked to stronger immune responsiveness. Furthermore, testosterone, as well as adrenal hormones, have a suppressive effect on the immune system.[2]

Thus, it's not surprising that ADs primarily target females between the ages of 20 and 50, although newborns and the elderly may occasionally be affected. Overall, 75 percent of ADs occur in women. However, gender associations vary with different diseases. For instance, twenty times more women than men develop autoimmune thyroid disease, while only twice as many women as men develop MS. With the exception of ankylosing spondylitis, an AD that results in a crippling of the spine in primarily men, women outnumber men in almost every category of autoimmune disease.

In Graves' disease, although women are seven times more likely to be affected, men tend to develop symptoms at an older age than women.

And in the case of Graves' ophthalmopathy, the associated eye disorder, symptoms in men tend to be more severe.

Familial and Environmental Factors

Patients with a family history of AD are more likely than other individuals to be affected. Furthermore, patients with one AD are more likely than normal individuals to develop another AD. The results of many studies suggest that many, if not all, patients with ADs have more than one autoimmune disorder.

Demographics of disease vary among different geographic regions. For instance, because iodine can trigger autoimmune thyroid disease, the iodine content of different regions influences the prevalence of autoimmune thyroid disease in a particular region.

Pregnancy is known to induce the development of several different ADs. Researchers attribute this to fluctuating hormone levels and note that there is also a tendency for mothers to develop autoimmune disorders, especially thyroid disorders, during the postpartum period, within 6 months after delivery.

With the exception of SLE, most patients with an AD experience a reduction of symptoms during pregnancy because of the body's natural immune system suppression. This is a natural protective mechanism that keeps the mother from rejecting the fetus.

Ethnicity and Epidemiology

Race is a factor as well with some ADs occurring more frequently in certain minority populations. For example, SLE is more common in African-American and Hispanic women than in Caucasian women of European ancestry, whereas rheumatoid arthritis and scleroderma affect a higher percentage of residents in some Native American communities than in the general United States population.[3]

DIAGNOSTIC DIFFICULTIES

Difficulties in diagnosing ADs have been explored at Congressional Hearings on Health Reform. In 2000, Olympic athlete Gayle Devers testified that her Graves' disease diagnosis took two years, two years in which she suffered while her symptoms worsened. And most patients with ADs wait much longer before they're accurately diagnosed.

Predominant symptoms may also vary among age groups and in different populations, confusing diagnosis. As an example, in Graves' disease, an autoimmune hyperthyroid disorder, the most common symptoms seen in younger patients are nervousness and anxiety. However, in elderly Graves' patients, the primary symptoms often include apathy and depression, leading to the term "apathetic Graves' disease." Overall symptoms in Graves' disease also include elation, moodiness and weight loss, although weight gain is seen in 10 percent of Graves' patients.

OVERLAPPING SYMPTOMS

AD diagnosis is typically based on the presence of specific disease symptoms in combination with laboratory results, including the presence of immune system and genetic markers. Although many of the symptoms overlap, each specific autoimmune disease is associated with a specific cluster of symptoms and abnormal laboratory results.

For instance, in many ADs, specific antibody tests can help with diagnosis. In SLE, for example, antinuclear antibodies (ANA) are typically present in high titers. However, ANA can also occur in patients with Sjögren's syndrome and rheumatoid arthritis. Further testing for double stranded (ds) DNA antibodies is helpful since (ds) DNA antibodies are usually seen in SLE, although they're negative in the other connective tissue disorders.

Antibody testing aids in diagnosis, but a positive test, as mentioned, doesn't necessarily confirm disease. And some AD patients may have negligible autoantibody titers. In gluten sensitivity enteropathy (GSE), which is also known as celiac disease, patients often have low levels of IgA. Consequently, they have negative results for the IgA gliadin antibodies associated with GSE. However, IgG antibodies are generally positive in these individuals unless they have already started a gluten free diet.

What Went Wrong?
The Players in
Autoimmune Disease

Returning to our ill-fated sandcastle and embellishing from a Taoist perspective, it's easy to understand how and why ADs develop. Taoism, after all, teaches us that everything in the universe is dynamic. Therefore, the relationship of one grain of sand to another or one cell to another is also a dynamic or constantly changing process.

For example, if the wind shifted only one grain of sand, this change would eventually cause other granules to shift. As each speck of sand shifted, other sections of the castle, even ones on the opposite side, would be affected. Similarly, every bit of food we ingest, every emotion we feel, and even the air we breathe all influence other bodily systems, including the immune system.

This chapter describes the dynamic workings of the immune system. Specifically, it explains how the immune system cells produce auto-antibodies and cause inflammation, and it explains how these changes lead to the development of autoimmune disease.

HOMEOSTASIS

The body's major organs are like the windows and steeples of our sandcastle. As Taoism teaches, changes affecting specific organs or specific parts of the castle directly influence other organs or other castle components. For instance, in insulin dependent diabetes mellitus, autoantibodies produced by the immune system cells attack islet cells in the pancreas, destroying these cells.

Normally, pancreatic islet cells produce and release insulin, a hormone that regulates blood sugar levels, keeping them from rising too high. As a consequence of having destroyed islet cells, insulin levels decline. And consequently, the blood sugar or glucose level soars. The high blood sugar level (hyperglycemia) damages other organs, mainly the kidneys and the nerves. Impaired kidney function, in turn, can affect the heart, and disturbed heart function can compromise the lungs. And so on.

While our sandcastle gracefully surrenders to its granular collapse, the cells of the human body face catastrophe by rushing to the rescue. In a process known as homeostasis, cells throughout the body join together in an effort to maintain health. For instance, responding to the increased blood nitrogen levels that result when damaged kidneys can no longer filter waste effectively, muscle tissue cells release lactic acid in an attempt to maintain a normal acid-base balance, or pH. And white blood cells travel from blood and lymph nodes to the affected area in an effort to prevent infection.

Homeostasis is a term originally coined in 1935 by the Harvard physiologist Dr. Walter Cannon. An example of homeostasis is demonstrated by the immune response. In the immune response, white blood cells rush to the point of injury or foreign threat and multiply. In the process they also release various protective chemicals that aid in healing.

Apoptosis

It would seem that this constant multiplying of cells during the immune response could result in cellular overload. However, each of the body's cells has a programmed time of cell death known as apoptosis. For instance, red blood cells have a life span of about 120 days, at which time they're removed from the circulation through the spleen or, in the case of large amounts of red cells, through the liver.

Apoptosis can be influenced by environmental factors, including changes in temperature. Alterations in apoptosis, such as the removal of lymphocytes before their time, can induce the cellular imbalances associated with ADs. Suppressor T cells that normally destroy autoreactive cells in the thymus are especially affected by apoptosis. The compensatory increase in parathyroid hormone associated with vitamin D deficiency, for instance, enhances T cell apoptosis in the thymus, leading to AD development.

The Stress Response

In the 1950s, the brilliant Austro-Hungarian chemist Hans Selye discovered the detrimental effects of stress on health. In experiments he conducted at McGill University in Montreal, Selye demonstrated that rats subjected to inescapable stress experienced a wasting syndrome similar to that which is seen today in patients with AIDS. In this syndrome, the animal loses both body mass and hair, develops diarrhea and commonly succumbs to a devastating infection as its immune system fails.

Stress is caused by change, and change may not always be adverse. In our response to stress, our brain's hypothalamus orders the release of two stress hormones, corticotrophin releasing hormone (CRH) and adrenaline. CRH causes the pituitary gland to release adrenocorticotrophic hormone (ACTH). ACTH causes the adrenal gland to release cortisol.

As a result of these hormones, blood platelets aggregate to help the clotting mechanism, preventing massive blood loss. Also, immune cells activate, and blood sugar rushes to muscles. Heart rate also increases and blood pressure rises. And cortisol levels begin their decline.

However, with repeated or chronic stress, this system becomes ineffective. It begins to take short cuts. For instance, cortisol levels remain elevated. Unable to respond properly, the glands send out inflammatory cytokines, particularly interleukin-2 and interferon-gamma. In many autoimmune diseases, including autoimmune thyroid disease, levels of these cytokines are higher than those seen in the normal population.

Calciphylaxis

In rodents, the chronic stress reaction eventually culminates in a fatal reaction characterized by calciphylaxis. In calciphylaxis, massive deposits of calcium accumulate in the skin and body organs. In his original studies, at autopsy, Selye found that the animals that died from experimentally induced stress showed signs of endocrine and immune system failure, evidenced by their atrophied glands and immune system organs.

Stress Reduction

The implications of Selye's experiment led to a new way of looking at disease development and treatment. A few years after Selye's studies were published, Dr. Norman Cousins successfully treated his own autoimmune arthritic condition of ankylosing spondylitis with stress reduction.

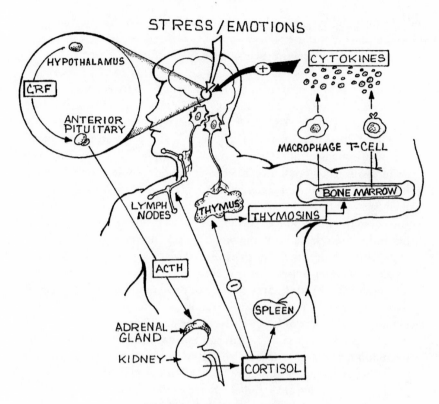

The Mind-Body Connection

Primarily using biofeedback and humor, Cousins achieved a successful long-term remission.

Although Selye introduced the circumstantial link and Cousins proved how reversing the circumstances could alter the consequences, it was years before researchers understood how chronic stress, both physiological and physical stress, damages health. Stress, for instance, causes immune system changes that lead to AD.

THE BODY'S NETWORK SYSTEM

This understanding came with the discovery of the body's network system and the realization that neuroendocrine cells exist in all three systems. Before this realization, the endocrine system, the nervous system and the immune system were thought to be separate entities having no influence on one another. Now we know that these three systems synchronize their efforts, with each system affecting the others.

1. **The nervous system** transmits electrochemical signals back and forth between the brain and the tissues of various organs via chemicals known as neurotransmitters and peptides that travel between reflex circuits. The nervous system may also transmit signals between tissues of one organ to tissues of another organ. For example, when you burn your finger, pain receptors send signals to your brain. When your brain registers the message, you experience pain. The nervous system relays its messages instantly through impulses traveling across neurons. The nervous system also produces substances that do not act across synapses, but rather are released into the bloodstream and travel to distant target cells. For instance, the hypothalamic-releasing factors that control the secretion of anterior pituitary hormone travel directly to pituitary cells.[1]

2. **The endocrine system** contains the body's major glands, including the thyroid, adrenals, parathyroids, pituitary, ovaries and testes, thymus, pineal, and the Islet of Langerhans in the pancreas. These are all ductless glands, meaning they release their hormones directly into the blood circulation. Hormones react with cell receptors throughout the body, causing changes away from these glands. For example, thyroid hormone produced in the thyroid gland circulates to the brain, where it activates receptors which influence mood and emotions. Because hormones must travel through blood and lymphatic fluid to reach their target cells, their responses are slower than neural reactions. The glands also contain neurosecretory cells that can act directly on the nervous system.

3. **The immune system** distinguishes self from non-self, and it protects the body against foreign threats. In response to bodily threats, some people flee and some fight back. Immune system cells primarily respond by fighting back—producing antibodies directed against foreign substances. When the nervous system and the endocrine system perceive stress, both physical and psychological stress, they communicate this to the immune system, causing changes in immune system cells. With chronic stress, over time, these changes can damage the immune system.

Hormones

Hormones are chemicals released by glands into the bloodstream, and transported to a distant or trophic organ to exert specific actions. Recently, it's been found that hormones can also act on contiguous or neighbor cells, producing a *paracrine* effect. Hormones can also modify the secretory activity of the cells that produce them, producing an *autocrine* effect. In performing their autocrine functions, hormones aren't released into the bloodstream. However, they still exert action typical of their hormonal nature by binding to specific cell receptors.

Hormones fall into three general categories. (1) Hormones derived from single amino acids are called amines and include norepinephrine, epinephrine, dopamine and thyroid hormones. (2) Hormones composed of peptides and proteins include thyrotropin releasing hormone and growth hormone. (3) Steroid hormones are derived from cholesterol and can be divided into two groups: those with an intact steroid nucleus such as the gonadal and adrenal steroids, and those with a broken steroid nucleus, such as vitamin D and its metabolites.

Neuroendocrine Cells

The study of the relationship between the nervous, immune and endocrine systems is called psychoneuroimmunology (PNI). The nervous system releases chemicals known as neurotransmitters which can act as circulating hormones. Neuroendocrine cells scattered throughout the body, especially the intestines, also produce and release various endocrine hormones and catecholamines.

Several types of neuroendocrine cells also have receptors for hormones and neurotransmitters, illustrating their involvement in the body's network system. Furthermore, certain endocrine hormones act as mediators within the central nervous system. Immune system cells have receptors for neurotransmitters such as endorphins, enabling them to respond to directives from both the endocrine and nervous systems.[2]

The Body's Axis Networks

Many of the body's systems work in tandem to facilitate homeostasis. Acting as chief commander, the hypothalamus in the brain oversees and regulates pituitary, adrenal, immune and thyroid function. The most well known example of the neuroendocrine-immune system relationship is that of the immune-hypothalamic-pituitary-adrenal axis. In this system, immune system chemical messenger molecules known as cytokines, particularly interleukin-1, secreted during the stress response, act on the hypothalamus to stimulate the secretion of corticotrophin releasing hormone (CRH).

CRH, as mentioned, stimulates the pituitary gland to secrete adreno-corticotropin (ACTH). ACTH acts on the adrenal cortex to elicit glu-cocorticoid secretion. Glucocorticoids then promote the formation of neutrophils in the bone marrow and decrease the formation of immune system monocytes/macrophages and lymphocytes.[3]

Cytokine Influences

Immune system chemicals known as cytokines also depress the hypo-thalamic secretion of thyrotropin releasing hormone (TRH) as well as several pituitary hormones and neuroendocrine peptides, including somatostatin, thyroid stimulating hormone (TSH), and growth hormone. Cytokines can also elicit immunoglobulin production. Cytokines also directly regulate certain ovarian functions. And ovarian hormones, in turn, affect the immune system. The cytokine interleukin-1 (IL-1) inhibits progesterone secretion, and progesterone enhances the expression of the IL-1 gene in macrophages.[4]

Are You What You Eat?

Diet also influences immune system function. So does exercise, stress, aging, various medicines, sunlight, radiation, ozone and many other factors. Nutrients such as selenium, manganese, magnesium, copper, calcium, zinc and vitamin C are essential for the production of cer-tain immune cell components. Sugar and saturated fat have been found to adversely affect macrophage cells by altering their cellular mem-branes. This, in turn, reduces their sensitivity and effectiveness, depress-ing immunity.

Drug Influences

Certain drugs, including herbs, hormones and alcohol, also affect the immune system. Estrogen has been shown to cause a decline in T sup-pressor cells, making it a potential trigger for many different ADs. Specific drugs and hormones, which influence autoimmune disease development, are discussed in chapter 5.

Immune System Effects of Time and Aging

Time is an important immune system regulator. Immune function tends to ebb and flow according to the body's internal clock or circadian rhythm. Typically, the immune system is at its weakest at 1 A.M. and it peaks at 7 A.M. Levels of immune system cells and chemicals drop to their lowest point in the afternoon and early evening.[5]

The immune system also changes with age. For its first few months of life, the newborn is offered temporary protection by maternal antibodies. The human immune system is not fully developed until about age two. After about age sixty, immune powers begin to decline, causing a diminished, less effective immune response. Responses to autoantigens, including the body's own DNA, increase with age, evidenced by the increased rate of autoimmune diseases such as rheumatoid arthritis in the elderly.

THE IMMUNE SYSTEM TEAM

When we hear of the circulatory system, we can visualize the heart with its upper and lower chambers neatly linked to a system of arteries, capillaries and veins. But upon being asked to visualize the immune system, most people draw a blank. This is hardly surprising since the organs and cells of the immune system are scattered throughout the body and bear scant resemblance to one another.

The heart of the immune system is the bone marrow. White blood cells, especially lymphocytes, are its key players. The bone marrow, a pulpy, spongy tissue found inside bone, is the original birthplace of all blood cells and platelets. Distinct from red and white blood cells, platelets are blood components essential for normal blood clotting. The bone marrow also serves as the warehouse of the body's stem cell reserves.

Stem Cells

Stem cells are early or immature parent cells which, upon maturing, develop into one of the two different types of blood cell lines: (1) the lymphoid line, from which the white blood cells known as lymphocytes are derived; and (2) the myeloid or hematopoietic stem cell line. The hematopoietic stem cell line produces erythrocytes (red blood cells), monocytic and granulocytic white blood cells, and megarkaryocytes (platelets).

Stem cells have the ability to produce clones or, on demand, they can give rise to a different cell type. Recent studies have demonstrated the ability of stem cells to regenerate new liver and brain cells. During an immune response, the bone marrow produces clones of the specific lymphocytes needed to counter the antigen attack.

For instance, if the immune system perceives a threat from a type C virus, the lymphocytes with the closest receptor fit for these viral antigens will rush forward to initiate an immune response. These lymphocytes will also send messages via cytokines, telling the bone marrow to produce more cell clones to help with the immune response.

Bone Marrow Cells

While the bone marrow is responsible for producing and storing immune system cells, it directs these cells to the blood circulation and to other immune system organs as needed. Certain types of leukocytes known as T lymphocytes are sent to the thymus, an endocrine gland situated in the chest cavity, to mature. Thus, the thymus and the bone marrow are known as primary lymphoid tissue. The other immune system organs serve as storage warehouses for immune system cells and are known as secondary lymphoid tissue. Lymphocytes can originate in both primary and secondary lymphoid tissue.

Immune System Components

(1) Primary lymphoid organs, such as the bone marrow and thymus
(2) Secondary lymphoid tissue, including the spleen, tonsils, adenoids, appendix, lymph nodes, lymph fluid, the skin, and discrete clusters of immune system cells which line the urogenital and digestive systems; in the digestive system, which includes the entire alimentary tract, the most significant secondary lymphoid tissue is found in the Peyer's Patches, located in the intestines
(3) Immune system cells, primarily lymphocytes, macrophages and dendritic cells
(4) Powerful chemical and protein molecules such as complement and cytokines

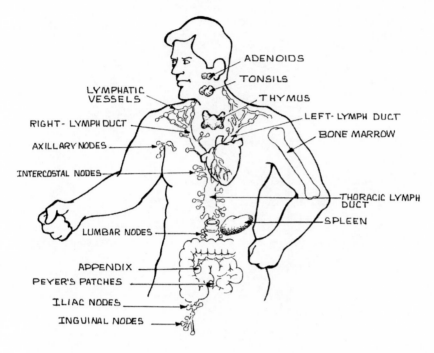

ADENOIDS

TONSILS

LYMPHATIC
VESSELS

THYMUS

RIGHT- LYMPH DUCT

LEFT- LYMPH DUCT

BONE MARROW

AXILLARY NODES

INTERCOSTAL NODES

THORACIC LYMPH
DUCT

SPLEEN

LUMBAR NODES

APPENDIX

PEYER'S PATCHES

ILIAC NODES

INGUINAL NODES

Immune System Organs

(5) Lymphatic system including lymph nodes, lymph fluid, and lymph vessels.

Bone Marrow and Blood

One of the major trains of immunology research revolves around the bone marrow and its warehouse of stem cells. At one time, scientists thought that all of these bone marrow cells developed into members of the hematopoietic cell system, that is, blood cells or platelets. Recent studies show that these immature primordial bone marrow stem cells are capable of maturing into other tissue cells, including liver and brain cells.

Stems cells can also be found in the breastbone or sternum, the skull, hips, specifically the ileac crest, the ribs and the spine. Stem cells are also found in the blood supplying the umbilical cord, which is known as cord blood. Smaller numbers of stem cells are rarely found in the peripheral (away from organs) blood circulation.

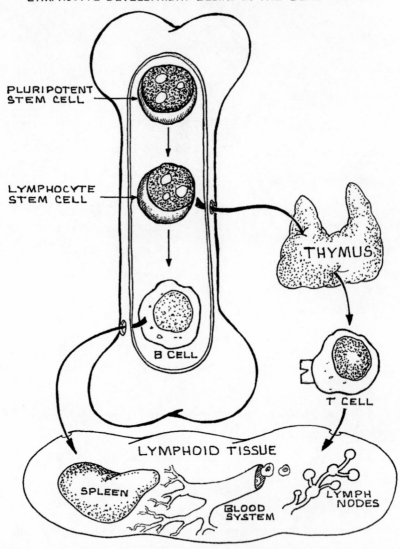

Primary Lymphoid Tissue

Blood Components

As improbable as it may seem, one minuscule drop of blood is loaded with thousands of different substances. The primary components include red blood cells and a smaller number of white blood cells. White blood cells (leukocytes) can be further differentiated into subtypes with their own specific immune system functions.1

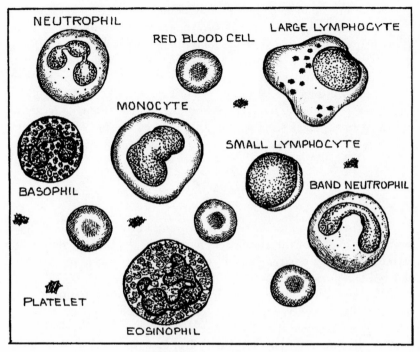

NORMAL PERIPHERAL BLOOD CELLS AND PLATELETS

Peripheral Blood Components

Leukocytes include macrophages, monocytes, granulocytes (also known as polymononuclear segmented cells or segs), neutrophils, eosinophils, basophils and lymphocytes. Usually, only mature developed cells circulate in the blood. However, in certain disease states early immature forms may be seen. Platelets (megakaryocytes), blood components essential for the normal clotting mechanism, also circulate freely throughout the blood.

Blood Component Autoantibodies

Autoantibodies may develop against both red blood cells and platelets. Platelet autoantibodies are primarily seen in idiopathic (autoimmune) thrombocytopenic purpura (ITP), a disorder characterized by deficient platelets, which causes abnormal bleeding and bruising tendencies. Red cell autoantibodies (agglutinins) are seen in autoimmune hemolytic anemia (AIHA), a type of anemia in which the body's own red cells are destroyed or lysed by autoantibodies.

Approximately 60 percent of blood consists of a liquid matter known as plasma or serum. Constituents found in this extracellular (outside of the cell) fluid include clotting factors, hormones, minerals, enzymes, ions, nitrogen compounds, glucose, proteins, and a number of other chemicals including the immune system chemicals known as complement and cytokines. The various immune system organs, which are described in the next sections, function to produce and store immune system cells.

The Thymus

The thymus is an endocrine gland found in the thorax in the front or anterior region of the chest cavity just below the thyroid gland. The thymus gradually enlarges during childhood and begins to shrink or undergo involution after puberty.

Although most blood cells and platelets develop in the bone marrow, a special subset of lymphocyte cells known as T lymphocytes travel to the thymus to mature. While serving as the site of T cell maturation, the thymus normally protects us from autoimmune disease development. In the thymus, virtually all of the precursors or parents of the cell lines programmed to become autoreactive are eliminated or made inert.[6]

During this process of maturation, T lymphocytes learn their true functions. Specifically, they develop the important attributes of self-tolerance and memory, and they learn to recognize the specific foreign antigen types they're programmed to defend against. The thymus also acts as a warehouse for other mature immune system cells such as lymphocytes, epithelial or tissue cells, macrophages, and other supporting cells.

Lymph Nodes

Most people are familiar with the lymph nodes that are located near the front sides of the neck. They may even recall occasions when these lymph nodes became swollen or sore, offering a glimpse of the immune system at work. After all, lymph nodes serve as ambush points for foreign antigens.

Ready to serve us during times of infection, lymph nodes store T lymphocyte cells and phagocytic (able to engulf infected cells) macrophage cells. Besides their immune system functions, these cells act as filters for particulate matter and infectious agents. Besides the cervical lymph nodes found in the neck, lymph nodes can also be found in the axillae or under-arm region, the stomach, the groin and in the para-aortic region surrounding the heart. Lymph nodes consist of three separate types of tissue clustered over sinus cavities and connected to a network of blood and lymphatic vessels.

The Spleen

The spleen is a muscular organ consisting of red and white pulp, which is located in the upper left quadrant of the abdomen. The spleen stores immune system cells in its white pulp and filters blood in its red pulp. The red pulp removes old or damaged red blood cells from the circulation whereas the white pulp acts much like the lymph nodes during an immune response.

Mucosa and Gut Associated Lymphoid Tissue (MALT and GALT)

Areas of lymphoid tissue are also concentrated in the moist mucous caverns of the gastrointestinal tract, the respiratory tract and the urogenital tract. Gut associated lymphoid tissue (GALT) is found in the tonsils, adenoids (Waldeyer's ring), Peyer's patches in the intestines, lymphoid aggregates located in the appendix and large intestine, and small lymphoid aggregates in the esophagus and the gut.

CELLS OF THE IMMUNE SYSTEM

The most important immune system cells are leukocytes, including neutrophils, macrophages and lymphocytes. Lymphocytes, particularly the subsets known as T and B cells and the natural killer (NK) cells, are the workhorses of the immune system.

T lymphocyte cells are programmed during their maturation in the thymus to react with only specific antigens. Some T cells watch for specific

MATURATION OF GRANULATED LEUKOCYTES

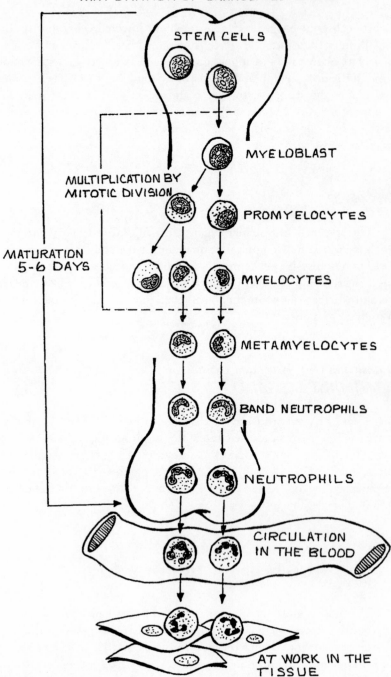

STEM CELLS

MYELOBLAST

MULTIPLICATION BY
MITOTIC DIVISION

PROMYELOCYTES

MATURATION
5-6 DAYS

MYELOCYTES

METAMYELOCYTES

BAND NEUTROPHILS

NEUTROPHILS

CIRCULATION
IN THE BLOOD

AT WORK IN THE
TISSUE

Granulocytic Cell Development

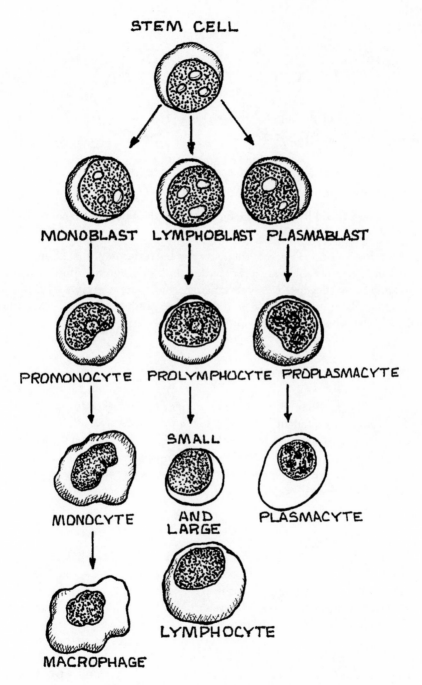

Lymphocyte Development

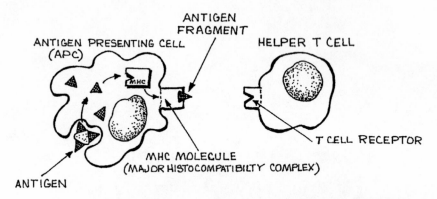

The Central Role of the Helper T Cell in the Immune Response

viruses while others are on the alert for bacteria or pollen. Since the immune system is able to react with thousands of different antigens, there are only a few of each T cell type hanging around at any given time. However, T cells have the ability to multiply and produce identical clones in response to attack by specific antigens.

T Lymphocytes (T Cells)

Anyone familiar with acquired immune deficiency syndrome (AIDS) knows how important it is to have adequate T cells. In AIDS, patients are deficient in T cells. Without sufficient T cells available to fight specific antigens, the body is said to be immuno-compromised. That is the weakened forces of the immune system enable the body to become host to a plethora of different organisms and tumors.

Types of T Cells

T lymphocytes have two major subclasses, the CD4 or helper T cells, and the CD8 or suppressor T cells. As their name implies, the T helper cells help to attack foreign antigens. In ADs T helper cells are usually increased, making the immune system aggressive. In addition, usually ADs are associated with a decreased number of healthy suppressor T cells, reducing the effectiveness of the body's normal protection against autoreactivity. T helper cells also have two subclasses, Th1 cells and Th2 cells, which help determine if the immune response will primarily involve cellular actions or if antibodies will be formed.

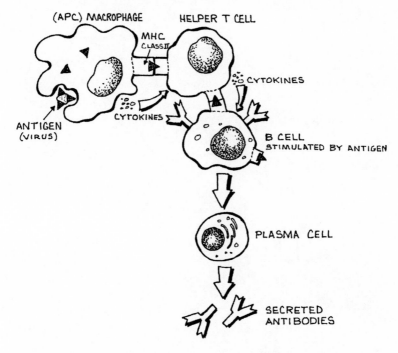

T Cell Response to Viral Antigen Leading to Autoantibody Production

Th1 and Th2 Subclasses

Th1 cytokines such as interleukin-2 and interferon-gamma predominate in organ specific autoimmune diseases. Cell-mediated immune responses, such as the tissue destruction caused by cytotoxic cells, represent the primary disease element. The autoimmune disease process is also hastened by the release of cytokines by or through antibodies targeting antigens on the cell surface.

Elevated levels of Th2 cytokines, such as interleukin-4, interleukin-5, and interleukin-10, characterize systemic autoimmune disorders. Other characteristics of autoimmune disease include widespread circulation of autoantibodies and immune complex deposits, and cell damage caused by complement-mediated lysis.

Cytotoxic Lymphocytes

T suppressor cells normally suppress or destroy infected cells, autoreactive cells, and tumor cells. In this capacity they are called cytotoxic

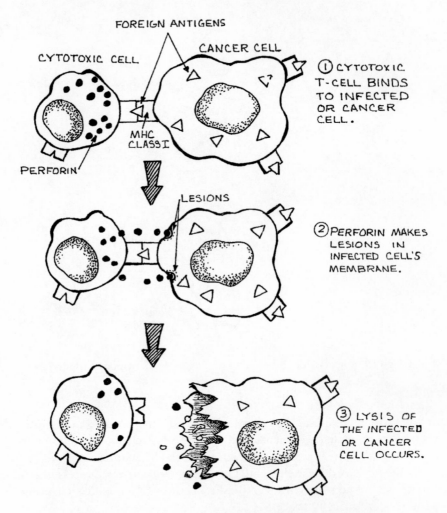

Cytotoxic T Cell Attacking Infected Cell or Cancer Cell

lymphocytes or CTLs. Other cytotoxic lymphocytes include NK cells and killer (K) cells. Because of this T cell dichotomy, people with T cell mediated ADs, especially autoimmune thyroid diseases, are cautioned to avoid immune stimulators such as the herbs echinacea and ashwaganda. Because immune system suppressants such as sugar and saturated fats cause a decline in already low T suppressor cells, they too should be avoided.

Recent studies show that in many ADs, including rheumatoid arthritis, the number of T suppressor cells may be adequate but the cells themselves are defective or prematurely aged, making them ineffective.

Furthermore, the chromatin in these cells appears to be damaged, although it's difficult to say if these changes initiated the disease process or occurred as a result of the disease.[7]

B Lymphocytes

B lymphocytes are responsible for antibody production. However, B cells only make antibodies when they receive the appropriate command signal from T cells. Once the T cell releases a specific cytokine that functions to alert the B cells, the B cell is able to develop into an immunoglobulin rich plasma cell. Plasma cells produce unique antibodies that target specific antigens. B lymphocytes are increased in many ADs. This natural increase is thought to contribute to AD development.

Lymphatics

Lymphocytes and other white blood cells also travel between other cells and organs, including lymph nodes, while suspended in a thick solution known as lymph. Lymph fluid circulates via lymph vessels. Lymph vessels channel lymph fluid throughout the body in a system known as the lymphatic system.

Cytokines

Cytokines are hormone-like proteins released by cytotoxic lymphocytes, macrophages and neutrophils. Cytokines act as immune system messenger molecules, regulating the intensity of the immune response. When cytokines were first discovered, it was thought that they were only produced by lymphocytes. Therefore, cytokines are sometimes also called lymphokines or chemokines. Cytokines aid in the healing process by causing inflammation and fever and they contribute to autoimmunity when they perpetuate cell destruction.

Cytokines allow immune system cells and organs to communicate with one another, and they determine the intensity of a particular immune response. Because of their ability to induce and prolong inflammation, cytokines are also responsible for many of the adverse autoimmune disease symptoms.

Cytokines include growth factors, interferons (IFNs), which are substances that help to destroy viruses, interleukin (IL) compounds and erythropoietin, which stimulates the growth of red blood cells. Cytokines that play major roles in ADs include:

• Lymphocyte activating factor (LAF or interleukin-1 {IL-1}), a compound required for the second step of T cell activation and the development of IL-2
• Interleukin-2 (IL-2), previously known as T lymphocyte growth factor
• Interleukin-4 (IL-4)
• Interleukin-5 (IL-5)
• Interleukin-10 (IL-10)
• Interleukin-12 (IL-12)
• Interferon-gamma (IFN-γ)
• Tumor necrosis factor-alpha (TNF-α), which promotes tumor growth
• Transforming growth factor-beta (TGF-β)

Each cytokine subtype has different targets and specific functions. Unlike hormones, cytokines affect organs and cells in their general vicinity. Of interest, some cytokines have different functions depending on the type of cells they come in contact with. And several different cytokines may cause similar results. With roles that both prevent and prolong AD, cytokines may influence both immune cells and non-immune system tissues to become activated, grow or die.

Cytokines and Symptoms

Many of the clinical and pathological features of rheumatoid arthritis (RA) are attributed to cytokines. Elevated levels of TNF-α, IL-1 and IL-6 are generally found in the joint (synovial) fluid of RA patients. All of these cytokines function as pyrogens, substances that cause fever and inflammation. Furthermore, in studies where IL-1 was injected into the knee joints of rabbits, symptoms of both chronic and acute joint inflammation (synovitis) occurred.[8]

Certain cytokines contribute to the thickening of the skin that occurs in scleroderma. Discovering which environmental compounds increase cytokine production helps determine disease etiology. Cytokines are used in the treatment of certain autoimmune diseases because of their ability to alter the immune response. However, they may trigger the development of other ADs. For instance, interferon therapy used in Hepatitis C and other disorders is associated with the development of insulin dependent diabetes mellitus.

THE IMMUNE RESPONSE

Tissue macrophages and other dendrites spearhead the initial immune response. By clustering or aggregating at the point of attack, they cause inflammation. Macrophages also have the ability to engulf bacteria and then destroy them by producing toxic molecules known as *reactive oxygen intermediate molecules.* However, if production of these toxic molecules persists unchecked, tissues surrounding the macrophages and neutrophils are also destroyed.

One example is Wegener's granulomatosis, an AD in which overactive macrophages and neutrophils invade blood vessels and then damage the vessels by producing these reactive molecules. These toxic molecules also contribute to inflammation in rheumatoid arthritis, which is observed as warmth and swelling. This inflammation also contributes to joint damage.

THE MAJOR HISTOCOMPATIBILITY COMPLEX

The major histocompatibility complex (MHC) refers to a group of immune system genes found on chromosome six. MHC genes encode proteins found on all cell surfaces, which subsequently act as immune system markers. MHC molecules determine which antigens one will react to as well as the severity of the response.

For instance, when a virus infects a cell, an MHC surface molecule binds to a piece of the viral antigen. Consequently, the MHC molecule and the foreign antigen form a complex known as an antigen presenting complex or APC. Certain cells are capable of presenting this complex to other cells. APCs are recognized by specific T cells, which have specific T cell receptors. Through this mechanism of antigen presentation, MHC molecules are important determinants of the immune response (see also chapter 4).

T Cells and the Secondary Immune Response

Before T cells can respond to cells bearing an antigen–MHC complex, another molecule on this antigen presenting complex must first send a second signal to the T cell. Cytokines act as messengers for this second signal. The relevance of cytokines to therapy revolves around the fact that

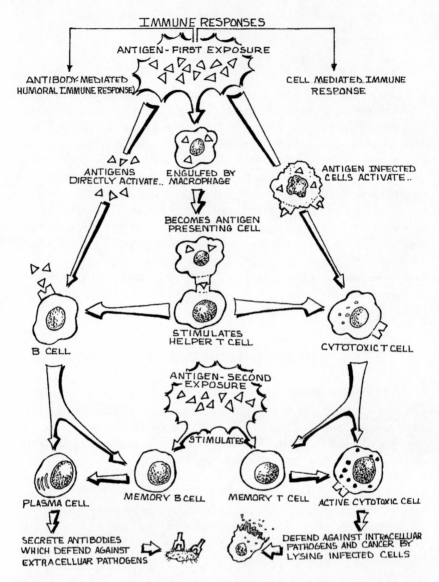

The Immune Response

if the cytokine messenger were somehow inactivated, the immune response would be altered, thereby preventing autoantibody development.

Natural Killer (NK) Cells

Natural killer cells belong to a specific class of lymphocytes distinctly different from T or B lymphocytes. NK cells are large granular cytotoxic (capable of destroying other cells) lymphocytes that directly destroy "foreign" cells. NK cells are capable of reacting without first becoming sensitized to a particular cell, making them valuable as a first line of defense. NK cells destroy other cells infected with viruses as well as autoreactive cells. In some ADs, such as Graves' disease, untreated patients have been found to have a decreased number of NK cells. This deficiency allows autoreactive cells to perpetuate, which, in turn, promotes autoantibody development.

INNATE AND ACQUIRED IMMUNITY

Infants are born with a simple immune system that fully develops within the first two years of life. In the meantime, maternal antibodies passively transferred through the placenta offer the newborn temporary disease protection. The ability of the immune system to protect against non-specific disease is known as innate or natural immunity.

As the body adapts to its environment and its immune cells acquire special functions such as memory, these cells produce antibodies in what is known as acquired or humoral immunity. Depending on the particular disorder, autoimmune diseases develop through an immune mechanism directly attributed to either innate or cell-mediated immunity, or to humoral immunity.

Effective treatment is directed at the primary mechanism. For instance, in autoimmune thyroid disease, a deficiency in T suppressor cells is considered responsible for autoantibody production.

Innate or Natural Immunity

Innate immune system cells are able to react with many organisms without first differentiating or targeting specific antigens. The innate immune system lacks memory and doesn't become more efficient on subsequent exposure to the same organisms.

Innate immunity refers to the initial immune response. Its role is to bar foreign organisms from entering the body and to attack those that enter. It prevents bodily entry through mechanical barriers such as skin, antibacterial substances and enzymes present in secretions, stomach acidity, coughing, sneezing, and vomiting, and the movement of fluids through the body known as peristalsis, which prevents stagnation or stasis.

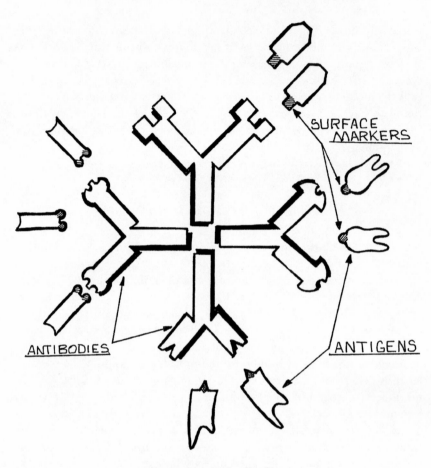

Antigens and Antibodies

Acquired or Humoral Immunity

As our immune system cells develop, a number of specialized T lymphocytes learn to recognize and remember specific antigens. Furthermore, they learn to produce antibodies against these antigens. This ability, known as acquired immunity, occurs in response to infection and other circumstances in which the immune system must adapt itself to react with previously unseen molecules.

The induction of immunity by infection or with a vaccine is called active immunity. When a non-immune individual receives serum or lymphocytes from an immune individual and is afforded immunity, this is called passive immunity. In this case, as well as in placental transfer of antibodies, the individual is receiving antibodies into his circulation directly instead of producing his own antibodies.

Antibodies

Antibodies are protein particles made from the body's immunoglobulin stores. Therefore, antibodies are also called immunoglobulins. When a particular antibody is directed against a self-component, for instance the thyroid, it's referred to as an autoantibody. Therefore, a thyroid antibody is also a thyroid autoantibody. In the immune response the body initially produces antibodies of the IgM class. It takes longer, generally a week, to produce IgG antibodies. Most autoantibodies are IgG antibodies.

Immunoglobulins

Antibodies are derived from protein known as immunoglobulin (Ig). The basic immunoglobulin unit consists of two light (L) and two heavy (H) polypeptide chains linked by disulfide bonds. Immunoglobulins also have an accessory J polypeptide chain, variable carbohydrate groups, constant and variable region domains and, in most instances, three different genetic markers. By varying a few basic ingredients, the body can produce millions of different antibody molecules.

Immunoglobulin Subclasses

Immunoglobulin subclasses include IgA, IgG, IgM, IgE and IgD. Among these classes, there are also subdivisions. Eighty percent of the body's antibodies, including most autoantibodies, are IgG antibodies. Only IgG antibodies can cross through the placental membrane.

In some diseases, such as SLE and Graves' disease, maternal IgG autoantibodies can cross the placental barrier, causing symptoms of transient disease in the newborn. However, immunoglobulins have short half-lives (time when the original amount is reduced by 50 percent), and the half life of IgG in blood is only 23 days.

WHAT DO ANTIBODIES DO ANYWAY?

Antibodies exist in two forms, either membrane bound, that is, clustered in tissue, or secreted, where they freely travel through the blood circulation. Antibodies have several distinct functions, the most common function being their ability to agglutinate or clump particulate matter including bacteria and viruses. Another function is opsonization, in which part of the antibody coats the bacteria, making it easy for cells to engulf it. Antibodies also neutralize toxins released by bacteria, for instance the tetanus toxin, and cause immobilization of bacteria. Antibodies that target the fine hair-like bacterial projections known as flagellae or cilae hinder bacterial movement. This prevents bacteria from moving away from phagocytic cells. Lastly, antibodies activate the release of complement, a chemical that facilitates the antibody's destructive role.

The Direct Attack

Acting directly, autoantibodies can injure intrinsic tissue. In anti-glomerular basement membrane (anti–GBM) renal disease, antibodies target fixed tissue antigens in the glomerular basement membrane of the kidney. Often the anti–GBM antibodies cross-react with the basement membranes of other bodily tissues, especially those in the lung alveoli, resulting in simultaneous lung and kidney lesions (Goodpasture's syndrome).

The Role of Complement and Immune Complexes in Disease Development

When antibodies are bound to antigens in the bloodstream, they often form a large lattice shaped circulating immune complex (CIC). When CICs accumulate, they often cause inflammation within blood vessels, blocking off nourishment to tissues. In the process of blocking blood flow, CICs ultimately destroy organs.

Complement molecules are proteins normally found in serum, the liquid portion of blood. There are more than 18 different types of complement (C1–C18) that circulate through the body in an inactive form. Like antibodies, complement reacts to the presence of foreign antigens. Unlike antibodies that attack specific antigens, complement proteins attack any particle lacking the appropriate self-marker.

The Complement Cascade

The release of complement molecules occurs in a series of steps known as a cascade. There are two pathways in which cascades are set in motion. Normally, protein molecules known as membrane cofactor protein (MCP) and decay accelerating factor (DAF) protect the body's cells from being attacked by the complement system. The normal function of complement is to aid in the removal of immune complexes.

However, defects in the complement cascade can hasten immune complex formation. For instance, in SLE, a C1 inhibitor deficiency is responsible for the destruction caused by CICs. Several other diseases, including arthritis and glomerulonephritis, result from the inappropriate deposition of immune complexes in the joints, heart valves or kidneys. A complement abnormality may be detected by screening for total serum complement activity (CH50) and determining levels of C3 and C4.

Immune Complex Triggers

The evocative antigens that induce the formation of immune complexes may be endogenous, that is, normal parts of the body. One example is the reaction to tissue antigens seen in the glomerulonephritis associated with SLE. Alternately the antigens may be exogenous, resulting from certain infections. Exogenous antigens implicated in SLE include bacterial products, particularly streptococci, the surface antigen of hepatitis B virus, hepatitis C virus antigen or RNA, various tumor antigens, *Treponema pallidum*, which causes syphilis, and *Plasmodium falciparum*, which causes malaria.

Regardless of the antigen source, antigen-antibody complexes are formed in the blood circulation. They are then trapped in tissue, for instance in the glomeruli of the kidney, where they produce injury, mainly by binding with complement. Electron microscopy reveals these immune complexes as clumps that lie between endothelial cells.

When the immune system's phagocytic cells eventually degrade immune complexes, inflammation subsides. Symptoms may also subside when the inciting antigen is short lived, such as what's seen in most instances of streptococcal infection. However, if a continuous flow of antigens is present, repeated cycles of immune complex formation, deposition and injury may occur, leading to progressive glomerulonephritis.

WHAT CAUSES AUTOANTIBODY PRODUCTION?

Through various mechanisms described in the following section, the immune system sometimes errs, producing autoantibodies. The specific type of autoantibody that develops is primarily determined by genetic factors. A defect in CD4 T helper cells is common to almost all ADs. Usually, there is either a reduced number of CD4 T helper cells or a defect in their response mechanism. However, an exact mechanism for the development of all autoantibodies is unknown. Rather, there appears to be several scenarios that fit. One of the most attractive ideas is molecular mimicry, where certain antigens have the ability to cross-react with certain of the body's self-antigens.

Molecular Mimicry

Immune system cells that fight bacteria can also attack normal cells that are carrying a specific mimicking molecule. Furthermore, if an individual was previously infected with the infectious agent, cells that were not initially affected are most likely to join in the attack. Cells injured by irradiation, environmental toxins or the body's stress chemicals are also the cells most likely to be tricked my mimicking molecules.

Infectious Agents

In one study involving *Salmonella*, a species of bacteria often responsible for food poisoning, it was shown that as many as 10 percent of infected individuals develop a reactive type of arthritis that persists for several weeks. But a smaller number of these patients develop a severe, long-lasting, debilitating type of arthritis. These are thought to be individuals who were previously infected with mild symptoms.[9]

Superantigens

Alternately, infectious agents may initiate autoimmunity by producing a select group of antigens known as superantigens. Superantigens include a number of different antigens, including particles of bacteria, which are capable of binding to a wide variety of T cell receptors. Unlike most antigens, which are capable of binding with 1 in 50,000 lymphocytes, superantigens are able to bind with 1 in every 50 lymphocytes.[10] Superantigens accomplish this by serving as a molecular bridge between antigen presenting cells and special binding sites on responsive lymphocytes.

Superantigens are potent T cell stimulatory molecules that bind to genetic markers, specifically the MHC class II molecules (see chapter 4). Superantigens are abundant in nature and are found on the surface of certain staphylococcal, streptococcal, and mycoplasmal bacteria or their toxins and on stressed cells throughout the body.

Factors Causing Autoreactive T Cells

The immune system mechanism in AD involves T cells that proliferate, producing clones in response to environmental triggers. During this rapid multiplication some cells become autoreactive. Factors causing autoreactive cell development include:

1. Alterations in normal immune cells by the type C viruses (oncovirus groups such as the California encephalitis virus) and retroviruses.
2. Haptens or antigens, such as androgens or endocrine disruptors, which may form complexes with tissue proteins.
3. Cross reactivity of foreign antigens; molecular mimicry.
4. Depression of suppressor CD8 T cell activity caused by HLA gene products which resemble the infective agent causing cross-tolerance with the similar agent. Furthermore, there are genetic influences, for example, normal people with HLA-DR3 genes have reduced T cell suppressor activity compared to subjects without HLA-DR3.
5. Environmental triggers including estrogens, viruses, chemicals, stress, ultraviolet radiation, superantigens, heavy metals, interferons and interleukins used in therapy, and heat shock proteins (also see chapter 5).
6. Exogenous substances, including injury or trauma, and dietary factors are related to AD development. The autoimmune eye disorder uveitis often occurs after eye injury. States of starvation, both by dieting or enforced in prison camps, have been known to trigger the development of Graves' disease.
7. According to one theory, autoreactive cells may actually be defective cells that are in the process of transforming into cancer cells. By signaling danger to the immune system, these cells, which show signs of premature aging, have the ability to follow a different path. By reversing their course of action, these cells conform to the process leading to autoantibody production rather than cancer.[11]

Why Me? Genetic Factors

Why do some of us develop autoimmune disorders when others with the same, or less wholesome, lifestyle factors and environmental exposures don't? And why are women four times as likely to develop ADs as men? Could it be caused by exposure to estrogen, a known environmental trigger, or is it related to the chromosomal make-up of females? Chapter 4 tackles these questions and describes the immune system, organ specific and other genes associated with autoimmune disease.

GENES AND DISEASE

A complex set of genetic instructions, known as the human genome, is found in the nucleus and mitochondria of most all of the body's cells. This information is contained on 23 pairs of chromosomes. Chromosomes are composed of long threads of a chemical called deoxyribonucleic acid (DNA) coiled tightly inside the cell nucleus or mitochondria. Each chromosome contains thousands of genes arranged like beads on a string. Genes, in turn, are merely segments of double stranded DNA that hold instructions for making specific protein molecules, such as those that determine eye color.

If the DNA language or code of protein molecules becomes garbled, the cell may make the wrong protein or an inappropriate amount of the correct protein. These glitches may cause disease. Autoimmune diseases are caused by a combination of genes.

Proving a Genetic Link

How do we know that ADs are related to genes and are not merely caused by chance? There are specific guidelines for establishing a genetic disease association. These guidelines include family clustering, studies of twins, and the demonstration of certain genetic markers. Unlike definitive genetic diseases like sickle cell anemia, where certain genes cause the traits linked to disease, autoimmune diseases are associated with a number of genes that confer susceptibility.

Family Clustering

In family clustering, certain diseases are seen more often in family groups than in the general population. For instance, 15 percent of Graves' disease patients have relatives with the same disorder.[1] Siblings and offspring of patients with multiple sclerosis (MS) have a greater chance of developing MS than non-relatives.

Twin Studies

In disorders with a genetic component, the incidence of disease is more frequent in identical twins than in fraternal twins since identical twins have the same genetic makeup. And the incidence of AD is indeed higher in identical twins. In cases where one identical twin has multiple sclerosis, the other twin is four times as likely to develop MS, whereas a fraternal twin only has a four percent chance of developing MS.

Genetic Markers

ADs are associated with certain immune system genes known as human leukocyte antigens or HLA markers, described in the next section. For instance, the majority of patients with Hashimoto's thyroiditis have the immune system antigen HLA DR5, whereas patients with Graves' disease are likely to have HLA B8 and HLA DR3 antigens. Occasionally, for instance in the case of the HLA B27 antigen, which is seen in 80 percent of patients with ankylosing spondylitis, these genetic markers can be used as a diagnostic tool. A negative test for HLA B27 in a patient with symptoms of arthritis can be useful in ruling out ankylosing spondylitis.

THE MHC AND HUMAN LEUKOCYTE ANTIGENS

The major histocompatibility complex (MHC) refers to the genes that regulate the immune system. These genes encode molecules that mark a cell as being "self" or part of the body. In man, these markers, which are found on the short arm of chromosome six, are known as human leukocyte antigens or HLA antigens. HLA antigens code for proteins expressed on the cell surface of all nucleated cells, especially lymphocytes. In other words, these protein markers, which are as distinct as blood type antigens, determine the cell's immune behavior.

Each person has two alleles for each of the HLA antigens. By testing for HLA antigens, scientists can find compatible organ donors (the body would react to tissue with foreign HLA antigens). And as mentioned, HLA markers can help diagnose certain autoimmune diseases. These antigens also help in establishing paternity since each parent contributes half of the HLA alleles to the genetic makeup of the offspring.

Testing for HLA Antigens

Most ADs are associated with more than one HLA antigen, and several different ADs may share a certain cluster of antigens. HLA B27, which is seen primarily in ankylosing spondylitis, is also seen in a number of different autoimmune rheumatological disorders. Furthermore, many of these genetic markers are present in 20 percent of the population overall, which means many people have these genes but never go on to develop ADs. Therefore, a positive test for an immune system antigen, in itself, cannot diagnose disease. There must be associated symptoms.

Of interest, different races are associated with different genetic disease markers. For instance, HLA DR3, DQA1 and B8 are associated with Graves' disease in Americans and Europeans, whereas in China, the incidence of HLA BW46 is increased in men (but not women) with Graves' disease. Since similar antigens are found among members of ethnic groups, some ethnic groups are more at risk of developing certain autoimmune diseases. Overall, Americans and Europeans are more likely to develop autoimmune diseases than individuals residing in other countries.

HLA Gene Classifications

Four types of HLA antigens exist, each of them having specific glycoprotein structure and functions: HLA-A, HLA-B, HLA-C, and HLA-D. The subset HLA-D includes DR, DP, and DQ molecules.

Within the complex of MHC or HLA genes, there are three subsets, Class I, Class II and Class III antigens. These different subsets also have different functions.

For example, Class I antigens are expressed on all nucleated cells and platelets. Their function is to alert T cells to the presence of infected or carcinogenic cells. Class I molecules are primarily responsible for binding short peptide fragments from self-proteins, intracellular microorganisms and parasites and viruses. (Note: Proteins are made of amino acids and linked amino acids are known as peptides.) Peptides bound to class I molecules are targets for cytotoxic T cells.

Class II antigens are expressed on macrophages, B lymphocytes, endothelial or tissue cells and activated T lymphocytes. Class II molecules are able to bind a slightly longer, more diverse group of peptides generated from extracellular proteins. The presence of HLA Class II molecules on target organs in patients with autoimmune disease is indicative of an autoimmune process. Peptides bound to Class II molecules trigger T helper cells that help regulate antibody production.

Class III antigens include several of the immune system chemicals, including complement and tumor necrosis factor (TNF).

As mentioned in the previous chapter, HLA molecules bind to antigen presenting complexes and help determine the type of antibody which will be produced. Class I antigens include HLA-A, B, and C molecules, whereas Class II antigens include HLA-DR, DP, and DQ markers.

Haplotypes as Disease Markers

HLA antigens determine which foreign antigens a person can respond to and how strongly. Furthermore, HLA antigens allow immune system cells to recognize and communicate with one another, resulting in a more active immune system.

Alleles are differing forms of the same gene that can occupy a given locus or position on a chromosome. The HLA system includes many closely linked genes, each having many alleles. When both parents contribute the same genetic marker (homozygous alleles), there is a stronger genetic influence.

The profile of HLA antigens or alleles that an individual has is known as a haplotype. Certain haplotypes associated with certain diseases appear to be inherited more frequently than would be seen by chance alone. This offshoot from chance is known as linkage disequilibrium and it facilitates the transmission of autoimmune diseases, explaining their prevalence in certain family and ethnic groups.

Haplotypes

The most striking haplotype associated with autoimmune disease involves the HLA markers A1, B8, and DR3. The frequency of this set is increased in patients with juvenile onset or type 1 diabetes, gluten sensitivity enteropathy, Graves' diseases, dermatitis herpetiformis, chronic active hepatitis and several other diseases.

Certain HLA antigens, including DR3, are associated with a decreased number of T suppressor cells, a factor known to enhance the development of AD. And certain HLA genes are associated with protection against specific ADs. That is, even when an individual has HLA genes associated with a specific disease, the presence of another gene, such as HLA B7 in Graves' disease, appears to offer protection from disease.

Relative Risk

Relative risk refers to the probability of developing a certain disease in the presence of certain genetic markers. For instance, patients who have the HLA DR5 antigen have a relative risk of 3.2 for developing Hashimoto's disease. That is, they are 3.2 times more likely to develop Hashimoto's disease than individuals without this genetic marker. That only a limited number of individuals with HLA markers actually develop autoimmune disease indicates the relevance of environmental factors.

The following table describes the relative risk of developing specific ADs when certain HLA antigens are present. Although space prohibits including all the HLA disease associations in Table 4-1, other HLA associations are interspersed throughout the text.

THE IMPORTANCE OF
HUMAN LEUKOCYTE ANTIGENS

When HLA antigens were discovered, they were thought to be specific disease indicators. However, we now know that in most ADs, the

Disease	HLA antigen	Relative Risk
Addison's disease	DR3	6.3
Goodpasture's syndrome	DR2	13.1
Graves' disease	DR3	3.7
Multiple Sclerosis	DR2	4.8
Myasthenia gravis	B8	4.4
Post-salmonella arthritis	B27	29.7
Post-shigella arthritis	B27	20.7
Psoriasis	Cw6	13.3
Reiter's disease	B27	37.0
Rheumatoid arthritis	DR4	5.8
Sjögren's Syndrome	DR3	9.7
Uveitis	B27	14.6

Table 4-1. Relative risk of developing specific diseases with specific HLA antigens. Most of these diseases have more than one HLA marker. Antigens listed are the ones showing the greatest relative risk.

role of HLA antigens is minor. Other organ specific genes work in conjunction with HLA genes. Furthermore, the protein transport genes that determine the type of immunoglobulins produced also play a role. So do T receptor and cytokine genes. The AARDA reports that genes account for approximately 50 percent of the chance of developing an autoimmune disease.

Autoimmune Diseases Associated with Human Leukocyte Antigens

From Table 4-1, we see that certain HLA antigens are associated with an increased risk of developing certain disorders. Certain HLA antigens bind tightly to both self and foreign antigens, causing greater genetic susceptibility. The DR4 subregion is associated with rheumatoid arthritis in many ethnic groups, including North American and Northern European caucasians, Japanese, Hispanic and North American blacks.

Type 1 diabetes (IDDM) is associated with HLA DR3 and DR4 antigens whereas SLE is related to HLA B8, DR2 and DR3. From these associations it's obvious that certain HLA markers cause susceptibility to

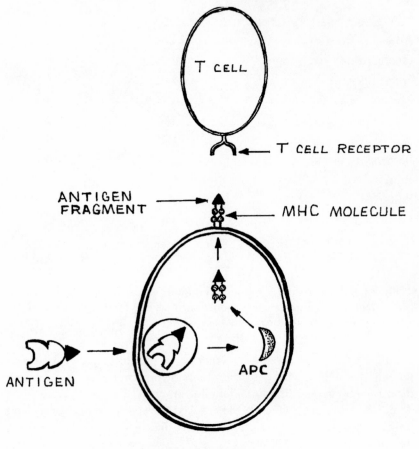

Antigen Presenting T Cell

more than one AD. This considerable overlap explains why patients with one AD are at risk of developing subsequent ADs.

The high relative risk of the HLA marker Cw6 for psoriasis seen in Table 4-1 accounts for its prevalence. An inflammatory and hyperproliferative skin disease, psoriasis affects about 2 percent of all Americans.

ORGAN SPECIFIC GENES

Besides the HLA genes, a number of other organ specific genes are associated with the development of AD. For instance, the autoimmune

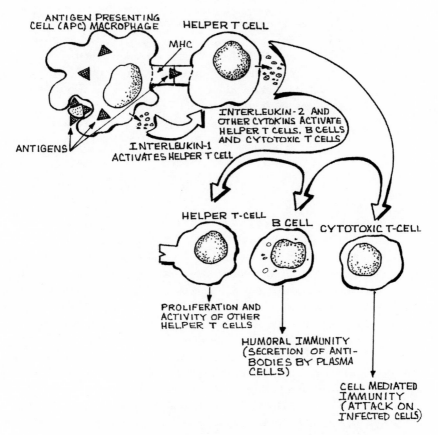

MHC-Antigen Complex Interacting with Helper T Cell

polyglandular syndrome known as polyendocrinopathy-candidiasis-ecto-
dermal dystrophy (APCED) syndrome is associated with the APCED
gene found on the long arm of chromosome 21. A Graves' disease gene
has been located on chromosome 20 and thyroid stimulating hormone
(TSH) receptor gene has been located on chromosome 14.

OTHER ASSOCIATED GENES

Because T cell receptors are programmed to recognize antigen/MHC
complexes and MHC genes confer AD risk, the T cell receptor genes are
thought to also be involved in AD development. As we learned in chapter 3,

T cells only recognize antigens when they're presented as an antigen presenting complex with MHC genes. This is known as MHC restriction. Furthermore, the HLA genes are known to affect AD development.

Receptor genes for various environmental agents may also influence metabolic changes that promote AD. For instance, individuals with polymorphisms in receptor genes to the aromatic hydrocarbons may be more susceptible to immune system influences of polyaromatic hydrocarbons.

SEX DIFFERENCES IN AUTOIMMUNE DISEASE

Most ADs are more prevalent in women than in men, which is hardly surprising since the immune response is typically more robust in women. The reasons for this sex bias are unclear but may include such factors as sex-related differences in immune responsiveness, response to infection, sex steroid effects with estrogen acting as an immune stimulant, and sex-linked genetic factors.

Dr. Yaron Tomer, Assistant Professor of Medicine at Mount Sinai School of Medicine in New York, has identified a marker for Graves' disease on the X chromosome, implying that a gene located there may influence disease susceptibility differences between women and men. In MS and SLE, some HLA class II alleles have been reported to be associated with disease more frequently in women than in men, which could involve changes due to the X chromosome.

Hormonal Influences

A great deal of research in this area has focused on MS, which is more common in women, although disease severity may be worse in men. All of the hormones studied, including estrogen, progesterone, growth hormone, prolactin, testosterone and DHEA are known to influence immune function, although not in the same way. For example, progesterone is known to inhibit certain types of T cell proliferation and to promote anti-inflammatory activity, whereas estrogen and prolactin stimulate T cell activity. Testosterone exerts a protective effect in many experimental autoimmune diseases.

Pregnancy affects many ADs. In MS, symptoms generally abate during pregnancy with a lower exacerbation rate during gestation. However, pre-pregnancy symptoms usually return immediately after delivery. In rheumatoid arthritis, patients often enter remission during pregnancy. In contrast, women with SLE do not improve during pregnancy, and many women (8 percent to 74 percent) report an exacerbation of symptoms. Some researchers feel this variability hinges on the patient's state immediately prior to conception.[2] The role of estrogen in triggering ADs is explored in the following chapter.

GENES REGULATING METABOLISM

Genes that regulate various metabolic processes are also associated with AD development. For instance, patients with celiac disease are known to have higher levels of the protein zonulin, which is under genetic control. And mice with a gene defect causing flawed carbohydrate metabolism develop a disorder similar to that of lupus in humans. Changes in glutamic acid decarboxylase expression or suppression in pancreatic beta cells are also associated with the development of Type 1 diabetes.

AUTOIMMUNITY AS A FORM OF NATURAL PROTECTION

The genes associated with autoimmunity are common and reported to be present in up to 20 percent of the population. Besides providing susceptibility to autoimmunity, they render a heightened immune response. According to some researchers, this suggests that these genes may have served some selective advantage during human evolution.

5

Environmental Triggers of Autoimmune Disease

A National Institutes of Health (NIH) publication, *Understanding Autoimmune Disease*, advises, "Patients should be monitored closely by their doctors so environmental factors or triggers that may worsen the disease can be discussed and avoided and new medical therapy can be started as soon as possible."[1]

Unfortunately, few patients ever hear this warning or learn about the effects of xenobiotics. Xenobiotics are foreign substances of synthetic, natural, or biologic origin that can affect the immune system (and other bodily systems) causing either immunosuppression or allergic and autoimmune responses.

In this chapter, I describe some suspected environmental triggers of autoimmune disease, including those discussed at the *Workshop Linking Environmental Agents to Autoimmune Diseases* held in September 1998 at Research Triangle Park, North Carolina. The National Institutes of Health along with the Environmental Protection Agency, AARDA and the Juvenile Diabetes Foundation International jointly sponsored this conference.

THE MAD HATTER'S
APPROACH TO THE ENVIRONMENT

As the Mad Hatter sadly learned, seemingly innocent environmental substances can cause a great deal of harm. Chemical regulatory agencies act much like the Mad Hatter in that they permit the introduction of thousands of new chemicals each year without any proof of safety.

As long as these chemicals don't cause obvious immediate damage, they're approved for release. As for their long-term immune system and endocrine effects, well, the burden of proof is often left to us, the consumer.

For example, the Environmental Protection Agency (EPA) has formally registered about 150 pesticides while thousands more are on the market awaiting review. In a May 1995 report to Congress, the General Accounting Office reported, "Most of these products may continue to be sold and distributed even though knowledge of their health and environmental effects is incomplete."[2]

In fact, scientists at the environmental conference at Research Triangle Park addressed the fact that there are no well-validated methods for assessing potential effects of chemical on the immune system. After all, how ethical is it to subject test and control groups to a potential hazard, then watch and wait for symptoms of autoimmune disease? In vitro (outside of the body) tests can be performed to assess these immune system changes, but up until now they haven't been.

And the enormous task of gauging what critical level of lifetime exposure might cause autoimmunity adds to the challenge, especially considering the genetic differences that make only some of us susceptible to developing these diseases.

Conference attendees concluded that the state of the science with respect to environmental agents and ADs is in the early stages of hazard identification. Although there is a wealth of compelling anecdotal and statistical evidence along with a scattering of animal studies, there are few peer-reviewed double blind studies (see also chapter 10).

METALS AND MINERALS

Mercury, Cadmium and Lead

The earth's core contains scattered deposits of mercury. In its crude sulfide form it is known as cinnabar. Mining and coal burning release appreciable levels of mercury into the biosphere and atmosphere. Everyday sources of mercury include fluorescent lights, batteries, thermometers, electronic devices, and medical compounds including vaccines and dental amalgam. Mercury released from amalgam fillings is the major source of human exposure to mercury vapor. From fillings, mercury can spread into surrounding tissue and cause symptoms of MS.[3]

Medicine and Mercury

Although the use of mercury in medicine has declined in recent years, the risk of mercury induced AD persists because mercury is currently used as a preservative in some immunoglobulin and vaccine preparations and can also occur as a contaminant of fish, imported food supplements and unregulated health products.[4]

Thimerosal, the mercury preservative in vaccines, is slowly being phased out. In 1999 the Food and Drug Administration acknowledged that vaccines expose infants to levels of mercury considered unsafe by the EPA. And there is a link between mercury and both autoimmunity and neurotoxicity.[5] There are also increasing reports of autoimmune myofascitis occurring from hepatitis and tetanus vaccines containing thimerosal.[6]

Another recent report describes 5 patients who developed SLE shortly after immunizations and concludes that epidemiological studies need to be performed to examine this association in more detail.[7]

Mercury Madness

Although it has long been associated with AD development, in the early 1900s mercury was commonly used in medications, especially diuretics, laxatives, skin ointments and fungicides. Nearly a century ago, in South Africa, epidemics of autoimmune kidney disease occurred as a result of mercury-based skin bleaching products. Mercury induces antinuclear antibodies, scleroderma-like disease, lichen planus, and membranous nephropathy (kidney disease) in some patients.

Besides medical and cosmetic sources, mercury occurs as a contaminant in water due to industrial waste. This practice has been associated with devastating incidents of toxicity, the most notorious in Japan. In this incident, methyl mercury, a readily available toxic form of mercury, contaminated fish in this region, and the local population consumed the fish. Many people developed ADs. In addition to industry's contribution, mercury is also produced and released by certain forms of aquatic life.

Xenobiotic Effects

In the body, mercury forms compounds that easily cross the blood brain barrier, damaging brain cells. Mercury affects the amygdala, hippocampus, and cerebellum. The neurotoxicity caused by mercury parallels the changes seen in autism, suggesting a strong likelihood that mercury in vaccines is causing neurologic injury in children.[8]

When mercury attaches to protein molecules it forms compounds that are particularly toxic to kidney cells. In animal models, injections of mercuric chloride cause the productions of antibodies against the kidney's glomerular basement membrane. These autoantibodies cause immune deposits in the kidneys and excess protein in the urine.

Studies indicate that these autoantibodies target protein molecules outside of the cell matrix, including laminin, collagen, and fibronectin. Other AD symptoms include increased levels of immunoglobulins, antibodies to DNA and a Sjögren-like syndrome.[9]

Although occupational exposure to mercury doesn't usually result in autoimmune disease, there have been reports of workers exposed to mercury developing DNA autoantibodies. Mercury also inhibits the production of IFN-γ and it induces IL-4 synthesis. This influences Th cells to produce more Th2 cells, contributing to systemic autoimmunity. Mercury also decreases the potency of Natural Killer cells and induces the expression of heat shock proteins, described later in this chapter.[10]

Lead, Cadmium, Gold and Silver

In humans exposed to cadmium and gold, autoimmune responses and renal disease, similar to that seen with mercury, are often seen. In metal-induced AD, symptoms usually end after withdrawal of the metal. Lead and cadmium are also associated with the development of autoantibodies targeting the nervous system.

The medical literature contains numerous reports of ADs that are associated with gold preparations, including gold salts, folk remedies, and liquors. Although its use is no longer as extensive, since the 1920s gold compounds have been used for the treatment of arthritis. The therapeutic mechanism of gold is uncertain but is thought to stem from its ability to inhibit certain proinflammatory transcription factors.

Patients with rheumatoid arthritis using gold therapy have been shown to have antinuclear antibodies against the Ro antigens. Associated symptoms include severe skin eruptions, proteinuria (excess urinary protein), renal lesions, nephritic syndrome, leukopenia, Sjögren's syndrome, and thrombocytopenia (low platelet counts).

Silver has immunotoxic effects on human lymphocytes and neutrophils, but to date there have been no reports of kidney autoimmunity.

Iodine and Lithium

Iodine is the chief component of thyroid hormone, and it is essential for normal thyroid function. However, iodine is a trigger for autoimmune thyroid disease. Iodine supplementation in patients with endemic goiter induces thyroid autoantibodies. And white blood cells extracted from the blood of patients with thyroiditis proliferate when iodinated thyroglobulin is added to the solution.

Lithium is known to suppress thyroid function, acting much like an antithyroid drug. Lithium also exacerbates symptoms of hypothyroidism in patients with autoimmune hypothyroidism. However, on rare occasions, lithium has also been known to trigger the development of Graves' disease.

Silica

Silicon and oxygen are the two must abundant elements of the earth's crust. Silicon rarely occurs in elemental form. Rather, it binds with oxygen to form silica. Silicic acid is the major absorbable form of silica in man and has no known toxicity. Silicone refers to a family of man-made polymers containing silicon.

Freshly mined particulate silica can cause of lung disease (silicosis) in exposed individuals. Silica exposure risk is also associated with an increased incidence of both systemic and autoimmune diseases, including arthritis, SLE, scleroderma, nephropathy, proliferative glomerulonephritis and dermatomyositis.[11] In coal miners with circulating rheumatoid factor, rheumatoid pneumoconiosis (Caplan Syndrome) can occur.[12]

Silicone

In one recent study, it was reported that women with ruptured silicone gel breast implants may be at increased risk of fibromyalgia, a disorder suspected of having an autoimmune origin. The study, conducted by researchers from the Food and Drug Administration of the National Institutes of Health, found that when silicone spreads outside the border of scar tissue in the breast area, reports of fibromyalgia increased significantly.

The report, which was published in the Journal of Rheumatology, suggests that women with silicone implants should be checked to see if their implants have ruptured or if they have anti-polymer antibodies or antibodies to silicone in their circulation.[13]

Pristane and Mineral Oil

Pristane is a substance found in certain mineral oils derived from chlorophyll. Widely distributed in the environment, occurring in zoo plankton, various geologic sediments, and crude as well as marine and freshwater fish oils, pristane has long been found to cause symptoms of lupus in mice. Recent studies indicate that some, but not all mineral oils have the same effect. Human ingestion of mineral oil leads to partial absorption through the intestine. It is then transported to the portal lymph nodes where oil grandulomas form.

Inhalation of mineral oil or other hydrocarbons causes lipoid pneumonia and pulmonary lipogranumlomas, a condition once commonly seen in children until the Council on Pharmacy and Chemistry removed nasal inhalant preparations containing petrolatum from medication included in its list of "New and Official Remedies." The petrolatum in these substances was then replaced with saline.

Mineral oil and other paraffin compounds are widely used in medications such as laxatives, nose drops, vaccines, petroleum jelly, baby oils and as a coating for foods such as apples, cucumbers, and cheese. It is also used in the packaging of some dairy products including milk and in baked goods. The average American diet contains nearly 50 grams of mineral oil annually. This consumption is partially absorbed through the intestine where it is transferred by lymphocytes to lymph nodes.

Mineral oil, like pristane, can form oil granulomas. Pristane, however, is the only chemical that appears to cause a lupus syndrome (more typical than drug related lupus) complete with nephritis, serositis and arthritis as well as the characteristic lupus autoantibodies (anti-dsDNA, antiSm, antiribosomal P). The onset of pristane-induced lupus is triggered primarily by exposure to a chemical with genetic factors apparently controlling disease severity.[14]

Mineral oil's ability to cause AD in humans has not been widely studied, although hydrocarbon exposure has been linked to the development of Goodpasture syndrome.[15]

PARTICULATES

Particulate air pollution refers to an air-suspended mixture of solid and liquid particles that vary in size, composition and origin. There is increasing evidence linking atmospheric microparticles to ADs. Airborne particles enter as volatile gases (ozone, benzene), as liquid droplets (sulfuric acid, nitrogen dioxide), or as particulate matter (diesel exhaust, aromatic hydrocarbons, ground metal and mineral particles). In most instances, these particles must bind with protein molecules before they can evoke immune system responses.

Particulates suspected of triggering ADs include contaminants derived from the soil or atmosphere or formed in the intestinal lumen. Atmospheric sources include car exhaust fumes, industrial pollution and cigarette smoke. Antigen recognition and processing in the gastric mucosa may trigger autoimmune events.

Ionizing Radiation

Ionizing radiations are of two broad types: electromagnetic and particulate. Electromagnetic sources include x-rays and gamma rays. Particulate radiations consist of electrons, protons, neutrons, alpha particles, negative pi-mesons, heavy charged ions, and other atomic particles. Both types of ionizing radiation differ from other forms of radiant energy in that they are capable of disrupting the atoms and molecules on which they impinge. As a result, ionizing radiation produces ions and free radicals, molecules that cause biochemical lesions. Ionizing radiation has long been known to trigger SLE and exacerbate symptoms. Of the various sources of ionizing radiation to which members of the U.S. population are exposed, x-rays are the most significant source.

ULTRAVIOLET LIGHT, SUNLIGHT AND OZONE

Ultraviolet (UV) light and sunlight are known to exacerbate symptoms of SLE. UV light is also associated with immunosuppression. In mice, exposure to 300 nm of UV light results in the development of epidermal carcinoma. UVB exposure, besides being a known high risk factor for cancer, causes bacterial resistance. However, there is no clear evidence that UV light causes autoimmune disease in man.

In one recent study, patients with MS were assessed to see if exposure to residential and occupational solar radiation contributed to mortality. The study concluded that, unlike what is seen in skin cancer, there is a negative association with solar radiation and MS. Although symptoms in patients with SLE are aggravated by sunlight, there was no increase in mortality in MS patients subjected to increased amounts of sunlight.[16]

The pervasive air contaminant ozone is one of the most powerful oxidizing agents known. The major source of atmospheric ozone is from the use of petroleum products. Ozone damage appears to result from free radicals which alter the protein binding sites on DNA. Although ozone has long been suspected of acting as an autoimmune disease trigger, there is not enough evidence yet to establish this.

STRESS AND TRAUMA

Stress

Stress causes immune system defects that lead to the development of autoimmune disease. One of the earliest reports of Graves' disease involves a patient who developed the disease after being pushed down a flight of stairs while in a wheelchair. Certain ADs are also more prevalent in survivors of concentration camps.

Psychological stress may also exacerbate AD symptoms. The stress response ultimately leads to a depletion of the body's natural glucocorticoid stores. The remarkable benefits of glucocorticoid therapy in autoimmune disease caused early researchers, not understanding the hormonal changes induced by stress, to suspect that adrenal hormone insufficiency played a role in autoimmune disease development.

The Stress Response

The role of stress in autoimmune disease development is supported by recent studies showing that neuroendocrine activation and subsequent chemical and immune system imbalances occur in response to stress. Stress can activate the neuroendocrine and sympathetic nervous systems, eliciting a cascade of events known at the stress response, which ultimately leads to depletion of the body's natural glucocorticoid reserves.

This cascade of hormonal steps is designed to help us cope with environmental challenges. A defect in this mechanism, caused by stress induced chronic activation, results in imbalances of sex hormones, prolactin secretion, and neurotransmitters. These imbalances are suspected of contributing to the development of autoimmune and inflammatory disease.

Studies suggest that chronic exposure to stress can result in readjustments of central stress responsive neurotransmitters, chemicals that alter the hypothalamic-pituitary-adrenal axis. Chronic stress also reduces interferon levels. This limits the ability of NK cells to halt the autoreactive process. Also see chapter 9.

Physical Injury and Trauma

Physical injury, including that caused by extreme exercise, has the potential of inducing or exacerbating symptoms of AD in susceptible individuals. Injury to the eye has long been associated with the development of the autoimmune eye disease uveitis. Injury to the thyroid gland or even excess palpation can exacerbate symptoms of autoimmune thyroid disease. In fact, one Graves' disease patient in remission from antithyroid drugs reported having a relapse after her boyfriend attempted to strangle her.

Focal brain damage is suggested of causing an inflammatory response that may lead to MS or experimental autoimmune encephalitis. In addition, focal brain injury may reactivate autoimmune inflammation in patients already diagnosed with MS.

ENVIRONMENTAL CHEMICALS AND PESTICIDES

The years following World War II heralded an unprecedented influx of synthetic chemicals, advertised as better living through chemistry. The housewife spraying the most DDT was considered the cleanest woman on her block. However, DDT and similar chemicals degrade poorly. Extremely pervasive, they can be found in all parts of the world and in much of our food supply. Many chemical contaminants trigger endocrine and immune system dysfunction. In particular, polychlorinated biphenyls (PCBs) and dioxin have long been linked to the autoimmune condition non–Hodgkin's lymphoma.[17]

Solvents such as trichloroethylene, perchlorotethylene, benzene, xylene, and vinyl chloride used in the plastics industry and in solvent-oriented hobbies are all known to cause scleroderma after chronic exposure. Vinyl chloride exposure, which is known to affect individuals with HLA DR5 and induce the severest effects in individuals who also have

HLA DR8, is also linked to mixed connective tissue disease. Epoxy resin exposure has been found to cause a reversible sclerosis of the skin.

The artificial sweetener aspartame breaks down into methanol and formaldehyde, causing symptoms similar to those seen in MS. Aspartame is suspected of triggering SLE, MS and fibromyalgia. In one recent study of fibromyalgia patients, all women with multiple symptoms, all patients achieved remission after they eliminated the excitotoxins monosodium glutamate and aspartame from their diets. Excitotoxins are molecules that act as excitatory neurotransmitters, causing neurotoxicity when used in large amounts.[18]

Pesticides

Pesticides constitute an extremely diverse group of toxins including insecticides, fungicides, rodenticides, herbicides and algicides. Among the worst are the class of chemicals known as persistent organochlorine pollutants (POPs), such as dieldrin, lindane, the polychlorinated biphenyls (PCBs) and the potent insecticide dichlordiphenyl-trichlorethane (DDT). POPs have a tendency to lodge in our body's fat cells. And like aberrant genes, they're passed down from one generation to the next.

Having neglected to consider this, government inspectors were stymied in the early 1950s when levels of pesticide in baby food first exceeded safe standards. So they raised the standards, not realizing that these orphaned chemicals circulate through our blood, acting as endocrine disruptors, latching on to whatever cell receptors they can.

By binding to cell receptors, chemical contaminants block or mimic essential chemical signals, causing hormonal, central nervous system, and immune system imbalances. These imbalances lead to neurological, endocrine and autoimmune disorders. Besides disrupting the endocrine system, pesticides damage neuroendocrine cells in the nervous system, which, in turn, weakens the immune system.

Organophosphates

Furthermore, organophosphate pesticides inhibit acetylcholinesterase production. Consequently, the body becomes laden with accumulations of the enzyme acetylcholine. Acetylcholine binds to and stimulates muscarinic and nicotinic receptors found in autonomic ganglia, the central nervous system, heart, salivary glands, skeletal muscle and smooth muscles.

The brain is initially over-stimulated. Later, paralysis of neural transmission occurs and the immune system produces antibodies to the cytochrome P450 hepatic detoxification system.[19]

Dr. Warren Porter, researching pesticides and aggression at the University of Wisconsin in Madison, found that a combination of the weed killer atrazine and the fertilizer nitrate causes immune and endocrine effects, particularly thyroid dysfunction. [20]

Four years ago, Congress ordered the Environmental Protection Agency to assess more than 9,000 agricultural pesticides for their product safety. While progress in banning the most toxic pesticides is being made, a recent Consumer Union report showed that barely one third of the job is complete. Information on this study can be found at http://www.consumerunion.org, the Consumer Union web site.

Dioxin and PCBs

Dioxin or TCDD is a chemical contaminant that occurs as chlorine byproduct of the paper bleaching manufacturing process. Although it is useless on its own, dioxin is a common environmental contaminant. Dioxin was also released as a contaminant of the pesticide Agent Orange, which was used as a defoliant by U. S. forces in Vietnam. The highest concentrations of dioxin result from the incineration of medical waste.

Long-term effects of dioxin exposure on human immunity, reproduction and development remain the focus of ongoing research. One of the primary toxic effects of dioxin in laboratory animals is on the immune system, where even the smallest detectable concentrations cause immune system suppression or immune system overactivity, depending on other circumstances. The ability of dioxin to modulate stem cells and induce lymphocyte differentiation is mediated by the Ah receptor present in these cells.

PRENATAL EXPOSURE—
ARE THE UNBORN AT RISK?

Prenatal exposure to certain immunotoxic compounds may alter fetal development of immunity in mice, causing severe and sustained postnatal (after birth) immunosuppression in the absence of overt toxicity. For example, selective and persistent immune alterations have been observed in mice following gestational exposure to the organochlorine pesticide chlordane.

Other agents that injure the fetal immune system include hexachloroxyclohexane, DDT, polycyclic halogenated hydrocarbons such as TCDD, heavy metals such as cadmium and mercury, hormones such as diethylstilbesterol (DES), testosterone and cortisone, mycotoxins, and drugs such as acyclovir and cyclophosphamide. Several of the agents target the fetal thymus, causing thymic atrophy.[21]

DIABETES TRIGGERS

Besides viruses, there are three chemicals known to trigger insulin dependent or type 1 diabetes mellitus, two of which are prescription drugs. The cancer agent L-asparginase and also pentamadine, a drug used to treat pneumonia, and pyriminil, a type of rat poison, are known to trigger diabetes. All of these chemicals are capable of destroying the insulin-producing beta cells of the pancreas. Cold weather is also being investigated for its potential to trigger diabetes, and the protein in cow's milk is also suspected of causing the formation of antibodies to protein, which are suspected of having the ability to attack and destroy the protein component of pancreatic cells.[22]

POLYCYCLIC AROMATIC
HYDROCARBONS AND THE AH RECEPTOR

Polycyclic aromatic hydrocarbons (PAHs) are chemicals produced by forest fires, decay of organic matter, the burning of refuse and the burning of fossil fuels such as petroleum products and coal. Many of the PAHs, such as those found in coal tar, have been found to be carcinogens.

However, although there have been few studies of the immune system effects of PAHs, it's known that carcinogenic PAHs cause immune system changes. PAHs are also known to suppress cell-mediated and humoral immunity. There is evidence that the immunosuppressant effects of PAHs are due to certain of their metabolic products which bind to the Ah receptor inducing Ah gene complex activation. Response to the Ah receptor is under genetic control.

TOXIC OIL SYNDROME

In 1981, thousands of people in Spain ingested cooking oil that was accidentally contaminated with acetanalid or a related chemical. Some people died and many people developed a disorder called toxic oil syndrome. The acute phase of this disorder included pleuropneumonia and myalgia, and the chronic or long term effects included scleroderma-like skin changes, pulmonary hypertension, neuromyopathy and immune system changes including positive antinuclear antibody (ANA) titers.

PLANT PRODUCTS AND SUPPLEMENTS

Even natural products, including supplements, can trigger ADs. In 1974, supplements containing the amino acid tryptophan caused the AD known as eosinophilic fasciitis. This illness resembles scleroderma except that it is not associated with Raynaud's phenomenon, a disorder characterized by cold extremities. Eosinophilic fasciitis causes symmetric inflammation of the subcutaneous tissues, usually of the legs and arms, and rarely the trunk. A pronounced increase in a type of white blood cell known as an eosinophils (eosinophilia) is seen in the blood and affected tissues of patients who have this disorder.

Eosinophilic myalgia syndrome is a related disorder. Unlike eosinophilic fasciitis, however, eosinophilic myaligia does not respond well to corticosteroid treatment. Eosinophilic myalgia has also been traced to the ingestion of large doses of tryptophan. To this day, tryptophan is no longer sold as a health food product.

Canavanine

Canavanine is an analogue of the amino acid L-arginine produced naturally as a self-defense mechanism by plants to reduce their palatability. Dietary canavanine ingested through alfalfa has been implicated in SLE. Monkeys fed alfalfa seeds experimentally developed autoimmune hemolytic anemia, antibodies to double stranded (ds) DNA, immune complex mediated glomerulonephritis (the kidney disorder associated with SLE) and arteritis, an autoimmune disorder causing arterial inflammation.[23]

INFECTIOUS AGENTS AND VACCINES

Molecular mimicry and Superantigens

In chapter 3 we learned how viruses, bacteria and parasites can confuse the body by mimicking various self antigens. An alternative to molecular mimicry is the concept of superantigens, a group of organisms with similar molecular structures, causing crossreactivity. Regardless of the specific agent, certain autoimmune diseases increase during viral epidemics or after the institution of newly introduced or revamped vaccines. These responses probably occur naturally in most people, but for genetically predisposed individuals, infectious and toxic agents may initiate an autoimmune response.

Bacterial or viral triggers affect all ages. In fact, a middle-aged friend and co-worker was diagnosed with IDDM (juvenile diabetes) shortly after enduring a viral infection. He'd had his blood tested often in the past and had never had abnormal glucose levels. Having symptoms of persistent fatigue weeks after his viral infection, he ran a biochemical profile and found his blood sugar level to be ten times greater than normal.

One explanation for bacterial associated arthritis and other infection-induced autoimmune conditions involves the toxic waste produced by these organisms. Ankylosing spondylitis, in particular, is associated with bacterial waste in the digestive tract and colon. Mycoplasma, infectious agents resulting from a mutation in the bacteria Brucella, are also associated with ADs, particularly rheumatoid arthritis, chronic fatigue syndrome and fibromyalgia.

Studies show that many individuals with Graves' disease have antibodies to the intestinal bacteria *Yersinia* and also *Escherichia coli*, and individuals with MS have high levels of antibodies against measles, influenza C, herpes simplex and other viruses.

A Viral Link

Research done at Tulane University Medical Center in New Orleans suggests that several autoimmune disorders may be associated with a retroviral particle they're calling Human Intracisternal A-Type Particle or HIAP. Antibodies to these particles, suggesting previous retroviral infection, have been found in a very high percentage of patients with Graves' disease, SLE, Sjögren's syndrome, and juvenile rheumatoid arthritis. Researchers at Autoimmune Technologies in conjunction with Tulane

University believe that these disorders may result from the presence of HIAP in association with genetic factors and other external triggers.

Retroviruses

Retroviruses (RNA viruses) have the enzyme reverse transcriptase within their structure. This enzyme allows the virus to actually form strands of DNA capable of integrating with the DNA of host cells that it infects. Furthermore, some non-cancerous viruses have a tendency to exist as proviruses for long periods of time in cells without causing any apparent disease. In other words, they remain latent. An elevation of reverse transcriptase in the thyroid tissue of Graves' disease patients confirms the role of retroviruses as an environmental trigger in some instances of Graves' disease.

The SV 40 Virus

In the late 1950s and early 1960s, millions of people, including 9 million New Yorkers, were injected with polio vaccines containing simian virus 40 (SV-40) and other viruses. SV-40 was transferred from contaminated monkey kidney cells used to culture the vaccine. It is impossible to remove animal viruses from vaccine cultures. As a result of the SV contamination, many people have developed incurable ependymomas, mesothiliomas, and osteosarcomas that have SV-40 DNA as well as the whole virus embedded in the tumors. The recent detection of SV-40 in the semen of young adult males brings the safety of today's oral vaccines into question.[24]

Retroviral sequences (MRSV) have recently been identified in cell cultures taken from central nervous systems of patients with MS. Normally, these sequences would not be able to cross the blood brain barrier and enter the nervous system. However, adhesion molecules on cells and substances known as matrix metalloprotease enzymes allow activated lymphocytes access to the white matter surrounding axons in the nervous system. Activated lymphocyte complexes may contain retroviral particles.[25]

The HTLV-1 Retrovirus

Similar to the disease process seen in MS, the retrovirus HTLV-1 may trigger an inflammatory process in the white matter of the brain, which is known as HTLV-1 associated myelopathy (HAM) or tropical spastic paraparesis. The activated lymphocyte complexes in HAM cause lesions similar to those seen in MS.

Early studies on the migration of populations to Israel and South Africa suggest that exposure to something before the age of 16 years imparted a life-long influence on susceptibility to MS. Thus, by a process of molecular mimicry, viral particles with protein resembling myelin basic protein, can easily cause MS development.

Epstein-Barr virus, influenza, herpes viruses, papilloma virus, and certain bacteria, including *Pseudomonas* species, are all known to contain stretches of 4 to 6 amino acids resembling the protein composition of myelin basic protein.[26] Alternatively, superantigens, which are microbial toxins capable of stimulating whole populations of T cells, are capable of inducing relapses in animal models of MS. Superantigens can also stimulate myelin basic protein specific T cell clones.

Foodborne Pathogens

A recent report in the medical journal *Emerging Infectious Diseases* describes the role of the foodborne pathogen *Campylobacter jejuni*, which causes illnesses ranging from diarrhea to dysentery. Researchers at the Food and Drug Administration (FDA) found that up to 40 percent of patients with Guillain-Barré Syndrome have evidence of recent *Campylobacter* infection. *Campylobacter* is also associated with Reiter syndrome.

Campylobacter infections are also associated with stress. Normally, the immune system would destroy these organisms before infection set in. In 1 percent of patients infection with *C. jejuni*, the sterile post-infection process occurs 7 to 10 days after onset of diarrhea. Most *Campylobacter* infections are associated with poultry, sausage, undercooked chicken, raw and bottled milk, and contamination occurring from food preparation, particularly chicken, pork and barbecued foods.[27]

PANDAS

Pediatric autoimmune neuropsychiatric disorders associated with streptococcal infection (PANDAS) are one example of a disorder triggered by infection with an infectious agent. The organism responsible for this disorder is the group A beta hemolytic streptococcus. The disease process involves antibacterial antibodies that cross-react with brain components. Recent studies suggest that obsessive-compulsive disorders may occur in a subgroup of these children.

The Vaccine Controversy

Vaccines contain specially treated infectious organisms usually suspended in solutions containing formaldehyde, aluminum, mercury and tin. While vaccines have been long known to trigger certain autoimmune disorders, several recent studies show that both the infectious agents and the metals in vaccines act as environmental triggers of autoimmune disease, playing a bigger role than originally suspected.

After receiving a vaccine for Lyme disease, more than 70 plaintiffs involved in a class-action lawsuit developed symptoms of autoimmune arthritis including paralysis. The suit alleges that SmithKline Beecham, the manufacturer of the vaccine known as LYMErix, failed to warn doctors and the public that nearly a third of the general population is genetically predisposed to developing autoimmune arthritis and that LYMErix can trigger its development.[28]

More than 80 percent of children with autism have antibodies to myelin basic protein, the same antibodies seen in MS. In controlled studies, children who were not vaccinated do not show evidence of these antibodies. Dr. Edward Yazbak describes a study initiated in the U.K., Australia, and the U.S. designed to examine any connections between the administration of the measles, mumps and rubella (MMR) vaccine or any of its components to women in the postpartum period. Typically, women, often nursing mothers, with low or negative rubella titers are vaccinated postpartum despite the fact that recent studies show that the virus delivered via vaccines may be secreted in breast milk and transmitted to breast fed infants.[29]

Trials and Errors

In 1998 a French court ruled that SmithKline Beecham's hepatitis B vaccine, the first genetically engineered vaccine, had caused the development of MS in a child, prompting France to suspend compulsory hepatitis B vaccinations for schoolchildren.

Mandatory inoculations with the recent rotavirus vaccine, genetically engineered from a monkey-human hybrid virus, were suspended in the United States in 1999 after a significant number of inoculated infants suffered from life-threatening bowel blockages. Several recent incidences of autoimmune hemolytic anemia have also been linked to vaccines against diphtheria, pertussis and tetanus (DPT) and oral polio vaccines.

In Classen's study of the postnatal rubella virus given to mothers with low rubella titers after delivery, members of vaccine and parent groups were contacted via e-mail and given questionnaires to fill out. Over 280 replies were received within 120 days. These responses showed unexpected and alarming findings in 25 of these families, including the presence of the live attenuated rubella virus and the subsequent development of autism in nursing infants. That autism may be caused by an immune system response to a virus has been established since 1998.[30]

In another controversial report, health advocacy groups in the U.S. and Britain charged that public health officials in governments of both countries manipulated research data in June 1999 in an attempt to stifle further investigation in to the association between the live virus in the MMR vaccine and the development of autism.[31]

Furthermore, scientists at the International Public Conference on Vaccination 2000 expressed concern about a potential connection between autism and childhood vaccinations. The MMR vaccine is suspected of being responsible.[32] While vaccines are crucial for disease protection, the 39 vaccines routinely given to school age children are of concern, especially when homeopathic vaccines with dilute preparation of infectious agents are available.

Autoimmune-Autism Link

Dr. Anne M. Comi of John Hopkins Hospital reports that autism appears to be more common in families with a history of ADs, suggesting a shared genetic origin. Comi and other doctors advise that patients with a family history of ADs avoid multiple vaccines and not inoculate children who show signs of infection, such as a cold.

In May 2000, the FDA's Dr. Fred Miller told the Third Annual Conference on Vaccine Research held in Washington, D.C., that vaccines are safe, although he admitted that some ADs may be linked to vaccines. As examples he cited the link between arthritis and many vaccines, including the measles, mumps and rubella vaccine, as well as the link between Guillain-Barré Syndrome and certain vaccines.[33]

In another series of studies, the Institute of Medicine concluded that combination diphtheria-pertussis vaccines could cause Guillan-Barré Syndrome and death, the rubella vaccine could cause acute and chronic arthritis and the live measles and oral polio vaccines could cause viral infection, inducing autoimmunity.[34]

Adverse Vaccine Effects

A recent Government Accounting Office (GAO) evaluation of vaccine injury compensation noted that the worst adverse effects, including fatalities, occurred when children with symptoms of infection were vaccinated. Also, most adverse effects occurred within a certain timetable ranging from 24 hours to 30 days post dose, with most adverse effects occurring 3 days after vaccines. The GAO report noted that the timetable and the list of associated disorders had been reduced in February 1999, making the burden of proof for vaccine related injuries even more difficult.[35]

Heat Shock Proteins

Heat shock proteins are specific proteins synthesized in the living cells of both man and microbes as a response to heat shock and stress. Apparently a defense mechanism, this response is elicited by a variety of physical and chemical agents including heat shock, oxidizing agents, heavy metals, sulfur compounds, anoxia (deprivation of oxygen) and ethanol.[36] However, while cells are producing heat shock proteins (HSP), normal protein synthesis is impaired. Bacteria are capable of producing heat shock proteins that cross-react with cellular heat shock proteins. Although viruses don't appear to produce HSP, they evoke increased HSP production in their human host.

The expression of heat shock protein 72 has been demonstrated in thyroid tissue from patients with Graves' disease but not in tissue from normal subjects. This implies that Graves' disease is associated with an autoimmune response to HSP 72.

A Link to Atherosclerosis

There is significant evidence that the underlying mechanism for atherosclerosis revolves around an immune response to self antigens, particularly heat shock proteins 60/65. Antibodies to these proteins cause both atherosclerotic lesions and the buildup of plaque in blood vessels. In addition, elevations of MHC class II expression and increased cytokine levels have been found in atherosclerotic plaque. Coronary artery blockage is caused by a combination of inflammation, atherosclerosis and elevated cholesterol.

Increased levels of autoantibodies to heat shock proteins, gangliosides and oxidized low-density lipoproteins have been demonstrated in atheroslerotic lesions. The body's endogenous heat shock protein 60 that is expressed by endothelial cells stressed by hypertension, high cholesterol, components of cigarette smoke and other toxins may be mistaken for heat shock proteins produced by microbes.

Traces of Chlamydia and viruses, including Epstein-Barr virus and Cytomegalovirus, have also been documented in patients with atherosclerosis, supporting the role of infectious agents acting as environmental triggers. With atherosclerosis being a slow, complex process, it's likely that an infectious process is responsible for the initial disorder or that heat shock proteins produced by these organisms are responsible.

HORMONES

Estrogens

Overall, females have higher immunoglobulin levels, stronger immune responses, and increased resistance to certain infections. Females also have greater resistance to induced tolerance, increased ability to reject grafts, and increased CD4 helper to CD8 suppressor T cell ratios. Estrogens are the suspected cause.

Besides natural estrogens, humans and also animals are exposed to many environmental estrogens. Although the hormonal disruptor diethylstilbestrol (DES) is no longer widely used, it was once pervasive, occurring in milk products of livestock. DES is suspected of triggering autoimmune thyroid disease, especially in women who have DES induced vaginal changes.

Estrogen exposure can also be attributed to pesticides, industrial byproducts like dioxin, insecticides, fungicides, and herbicides that have estrogenic or antiestrogenic effects. Although these endocrine disruptors are not structurally similar to estrogen, they are able to bind with estrogen receptors, causing effects similar to those of estrogen. The list of endocrine disruptors is long and includes phthalates, the substance that makes plastics flexible, PCBs, dioxin and mycotoxins.

Studies show that while estrogen does indeed trigger autoimmune disease, the effects vary among the different diseases. For instance, during pregnancy patients with Graves' disease and MS usually experience reduced symptoms although they often experience heightened symptoms during the postpartum period. Patients with SLE, however, usually experience a worsening of symptoms throughout pregnancy.

Immune Effects of Estrogen

Studies presented at Research Triangle Park show that estrogens induce imbalances in T and B cells resulting in hyperactivity of B cells. Estrogen can either stimulate or suppress the immune system depending on dose, duration, site of activation and patient age.

In addition, studies showed that estrogen replacement therapy in postmenopausal women may increase the risk of developing SLE and scleroderma, whereas oral contraceptives aren't associated with SLE development. Testosterone is reported to have a protective effect on the immune system. Thymocytes, T cells, B cells, macrophages and endothelial cells express estrogen receptors. The addition of estrogen to these cells causes enhanced cancer gene expression, modified cytokine production, changes in immune cell apoptosis and changes to adhesion molecule expression, which may augment an immune response.[37]

DRUG INDUCED AUTOIMMUNE DISEASE

Many drugs trigger ADs. Substances with high iodine content such as iodine contrast dyes and the heart medication amiodarone can trigger autoimmune thyroid disease. Mercury compounds can trigger autoimmune kidney disorders. Substances contaminated with mercury and cadmium, including health food preparations and vaccines, can induce the production of autoantibodies to nervous system proteins. Furthermore, certain drugs such as quinine have long been known to cause autoimmune hemolytic anemia.

Drugs That Exacerbate Symptoms

Some drugs used as therapeutic agents for AD symptoms may worsen other symptoms. For instance, there have been several reports of the anticonvulsant medication carbamazepine (Tegretol) worsening symptoms of MS when prescribed to treat paroxysmal neurological symptoms and pain.[38]

Anti-malarial drugs used in connective tissue disorders may cause toxic effects to the eye. The first anti-malarial agent used, chloroquine, was found to accumulate in the layer between the retina and the sclera, causing destruction of the central retina and vision loss. Hydroxychloroquine (Plaquenil), one of the newer anti-malarial drugs, is not as toxic and vision loss is extremely rare, even with high doses. However, since

Drugs definitely associated with DRL.[a]

Chlorpromazine	Minocycline
Hydralazine	Procainamide
Isoniazid	Quinidine
Methyldopa	

Other drugs associated with DRL and currently in use.[b]

Acebutolol	Gold salts	Perphenazine
Acecainide	Griseofulvin	Phenelzene
Allopurinol	Guanoxan	Phenytoin
Aminoglutethimide	Ibuprofen	Prazosin
Amoproxan	Interferon-α	Primidone
Anthiomaline	Interferon-γ	Prindolol
Antitumor necrosis	Interleukin-2	Promethazine
factor-α	Labetalol	Propafenone
Atenolol	Leuprolide acetate	Prophythiouracil
Benoxaprofen	Levadopa	Propranolol
Captopril	Levomeprazone	Pyrathiazine
Carbamazepine	Lithium carbonate	Pyrithoxine
Chlorprothixene	Lovastatin	Quinine
Clorthalidone	Mephenytoin	Reserpine
Cimetidine	Methimazole	Spironolactone
Cinnarazine	Metroprolol	Streptomycin
Clonidine	Metrizamide	Sulfadimethoxine
Danazol	Minocycline	Sulfamethoxy
Diclofenac	Minoxidil	Sulfasalazine
1,2-Dimethyl-3-	Nalidixic acid	Sulindac
hydroxy pyride-4-1	Nitrofurantoin	Tetracyclines
Diphenylhydantoin	Oxyphenisatin	Tetrazine
Disopyriamide	Oxyprenolol	Thioridazide
Enalapril	p-Amino salicyclic acid	Timolol eyedrops
Estrogens	Penicillamine	Tolazamide
Ethosuximide	Penicillin	Tolmetin
Ethylphenacemide	Perazine	Trimethadione

Abbreviation: DRL, drug-related lupus. [a]Substantial observations and studies. [b]A few are single case reports but the majority represent good clinical observations. *Source:* Evelyn V. Hess (*Environmental Health Perspectives*, Vol. 107, Supplement 5, October 1999, p. 710).

Table 5-1. Drugs Associated with DRL

Features	Idiopathic SLE	DRL
Constitutional	40–85	40–50
Arthralgias/arthritis	75–95	80–95
Myalgias	40–80	35–57
Rash	50–70	0–30
Lymphadenopathy	23–67	<15
Pleurisy	42–60	0–52
Pleural effusion	16–20	0–33
Pulmonary infiltrates	0–10	5–40
Pericarditis	20–30	0–18
Hepatomegaly	10–31	0–25
Splenomegaly	9–46	0–20
Renal involvement	50	0–13 (hydralazine)
Neurologic involvement	25–70	0–2
Anemia	30–90	0–53
Leukopenia	35–66	0–33
Thrombocytopenia	20–50	0–10
Positive Coombs	18–30	0–23
Elevated ESR	50–75	60–93
Antinuclear antibodies	>95	100
Antibodies to histones	50–70	>95
Antibodies to dsDNA	50	<5
Anti-Sm antibodies	25	<5
Hypocomplementemia	40–65	0–25
Rheumatoid factor	25	20–40

Abbreviations: anti–Sm, anti–Smith; DRL, drug related lupus; dsDNA, double-stranded DNA; ESR, erythrocyte sedimentation rate; SLE, systemic lupus erythematosus. *Source:* Evelyn V. Hess (*Environmental Health Perspectives*, Vol. 107, Supplement 5, October 1999, p. 710).

Table 5-2. Frequency of clinical and laboratory features in idiopathic SLE and DRL

Hydrazines	Paraffin/silicone
Tartrazine	Mercury
Hair dyes	Cadmium
Chemicals used in computer manu-	Gold
facturing	L-Canavanine
? Trichloroethylene	Rapeseed oil, toxic oil syndrome
? Industrial emissions and hazard-	L-Tryptophan, eosinophilia myalgia
ous wastes	syndrome
Silica (quartz)	

Source: Evelyn V. Hess (*Environmental Health Perspectives*, Vol. 107, Supplement 5, October 1999, p. 710.

Table 5-3. Environmental factors reported to be associated with the development of autoantibodies and lupuslike syndromes.

vision problems may occur, patients on this drug should have periodic vision and field testing.

Drug Related Lupus

A number of drugs cause a transient lupus-like condition known as drug related lupus (DRL), a condition that generally resolves when the offending drug is discontinued.

Symptoms in DRL usually occur within the first four months of drug use, although they may occur after many years. Patients with both SLE and DRL usually have both antinuclear antibodies (ANA) and anti-histone antibodies. However patients with SLE have antibodies to double stranded (ds) DNA and patients with DRL only have antibodies to single stranded (ss) DNA. Patients with DRL usually develop symptoms of arthritis or dermopathy, but they rarely develop the nephritic syndrome associated with SLE.[39]

THE GREAT LAKES AND ENDOCRINE DISRUPTORS

The International Joint Commission on Great Lakes Water Quality targeted 11 of the most persistent toxic substances in the Great Lakes as critical contaminants. The list includes polychlorinated biphenyls (PCBs), dioxins, and furans; the organochlorine pesticides dichlordiphenyl trichlorethane (DDT) as well as its metabolite DDE, toxaphene, mirex, dieldrin, and hexachlorobenzene (HCB), the heavy metals methylmercury and alkylated lead, and benozpyrene, a member of a class of substances known as polycyclic aromatic hydrocarbons (PAHs).

Data on chemical concentrations in sediment cores indicate that the major loadings of persistent toxic chemicals to the Great Lakes took place between the 1950s and the early 1970s, with peak concentrations occurring in the mid–1970s. Studies conducted on human adipose tissue, breast milk and blood confirm that humans in the Great Lakes basin are exposed to persistent toxic chemicals through air, water and food. Limited data from epidemiologic studies conducted by the National Institute of Environmental Health Services suggest an association between human exposure to Great Lakes contaminants and clinical signs of immune dysfuction.[40]

ALLERGIES AND IGE

Recent studies have shown an association between allergies and autoimmune disease. Allergies have long been associated with increased levels of the immunoglobulin IgE. Furthermore, increased levels of IgE and also IL-13, a cytokine which is increased in allergies, have been detected in nearly 50 percent of patients with autoimmune disease. Several studies show that as IgE levels rise, symptoms worsen. In Japan, allergies to cedar pollen are thought to be one of the main causes of Graves' disease, and 10 percent of the Japanese population has these allergies. Graves' disease has also been reported to occur after severe attacks of allergic rhinitis.

FOOD AND WATER

While food and water are necessary for sustaining life, under certain circumstances, they can trigger autoimmune disease. More than 100 different pesticides are allowed in our food supply, and certain pesticides, particularly DDT, can disrupt immune function. And multiple pesticides cause a synergistic effect. That is, when more than one pesticide is present, the effects exceed the sum of the individual components.

Furthermore, as mentioned, food allergies trigger autoimmune disease. And some foods, such as gluten, can act as an environmental trigger. Chlorine and fluoride in our water supply can act as environmental triggers of autoimmune thyroid disease, and both of these compounds are known to exacerbate symptoms in patients with MS.

INTERFERON AND INTERLEUKIN

Recently, biologic agents, such as interferon, interferon-2 and anti-tumor necrosis factor-α, have been introduced as treatment agents for various diseases. The use of these agents has been linked to the development of autoantiboidies and autoimmune diseases, including autoimmune thyroid disease, autoimmune hemolytic anemia, autoimmune thrombocytopenia, lupus-like syndromes, pernicious anemia, and autoimmune vasculitis.

FETAL MICROCHIMERISM

In microchimerism, fetal cells are engrafted into maternal tissues where they continue to multiply and persist for many years. Recent studies have detected the presence of male fetal cells in mothers of sons up to 30 years later.

One recent study also demonstrated the presence of fetal cells in patients with Hashimoto's thyroiditis, suggesting that microchimerism may act as a trigger for autoimmune disease development.[41] In another similar study, nearly two thirds of patients with systemic sclerosis were reported to have microchimeric cells or microchimeric DNA, although 28 percent of normal (control) individuals also had microchimeric cells.[42]

6

Tricky Business, Diagnosing Autoimmune Disease

The AARDA reports that it takes an average of seven years and five doctors for most ADs to be correctly diagnosed. The typical waxing and waning of symptoms and the changing of predominant symptoms over time contribute to these difficulties. Furthermore, many symptoms typically seen in ADs may be entities in themselves.

For instance, many patients are treated for rashes, headaches, fatigue, hypertension, anxiety, depression, and arthritic symptoms long before ADs are suspected. Changes in insurance reimbursement in the last decade also contribute to the problem. Many insurance companies will not pay for diagnostic or screening tests, although once patients are diagnosed with an illness, they are eligible for these tests.

DIAGNOSTIC CRITERIA

Diagnosis is typically based on a combination of parameters, including physical examination, laboratory and imaging tests, biopsy studies, symptoms, family history, and response to treatment, with a favorable response to immunosuppressive agents suggesting immune system involvement. For some, but not all, ADs, a number of different established diagnostic criteria must be present before a diagnosis can be made. The following section describes diagnostic criteria for some of the rheumatic diseases.

However, most diseases are diagnosed, not by formal criteria, but on the basis of symptoms and immunological changes typically seen in these disorders. For instance, patients with progressive systemic sclerosis (PSS) exhibit dermal fibrosis (a process in which the skin becomes hard and fibrous, similar to scar tissue). Patients with PSS also develop skin thickening (scleroderma) along with progressive fibrosis of internal organs (gastrointestinal tract, kidneys, heart, lungs).

Furthermore, PSS is often associated with progressive lung fibrosis that results in diffuse pulmonary, interstitial and alveolar fibrosis. The remaining alveolar spaces are dilated, contain fluid, and are separated by septa and broad bands of dense fibrous tissue in a condition called "honeycomb" lung.

Sometimes, external appearance alone tips the diagnostic scale. In the advanced stage of scleroderma, the skin of the fingers exhibits a characteristic symmetrical tightening and thickening. This typically results in a shiny or waxy appearance and causes a tapering, claw-like deformity of the fingers and ulceration of the fingertips.

DIAGNOSTIC MARKERS

To help diagnose rheumatological disorders, the American College of Rheumatology has set standards for the diagnosis of most connective tissue or rheumatologic disorders. These standards take the typical symptom variability seen in autoimmune diseases into account. For instance, only four of the following eleven diagnostic markers must be met for a diagnosis of SLE.

Diagnostic Criteria for SLE

The 1982 Revised Criteria for the Classification of Systemic Lupus Erythematosus:

1. Malar rash: Fixed erythema, flat or raised, over the malar eminences (cheeks), tending to spare the nasolabial folds.
2. Discoid rash: Erythematous raised patches with adherent keratotic scaling and follicular plugging; atrophic scarring may occur in older lesions.
3. Photosensitivity: Skin rash resulting from pronounced reaction to sunlight, noted by patient history or physician observation.

4. Oral ulcers: Oral or nasopharyngeal ulceration, usually painless, observed by a physician.
5. Arthritis: Nonerosive arthritis involving two or more peripheral joints, characterized by tenderness, swelling or effusion.
6. Serositis: Pleuritis-convincing history or pleuritic pain or rub heard by a physician or evidence of pleural effusion; pericarditis-documented by an electrocardiogram or rub, or evidence of pericardial effusion.
7. Renal disorder: Persistent urinary protein greater than 0.5 grams/day or greater than 3+ on a urinalysis; presence of cellular casts in a microscopic examination of urine.
8. Neurologic disorder: Seizures in the absence of offending drugs or metabolic derangements such as uremia or electrolyte imbalance; psychosis in the absence of offending drugs or metabolic derangements.
9. Hematologic disorder: Any of the following—hemolytic anemia with reticulocytosis (increased production of red blood cells); leukopenia, with a white blood cell count of less than 4,000/mm on two or more occasions; lymphopenia, with a lymphocyte count less than 1,500/mm on two or more occasions, thrombocytopenia, with a platelet count less than 100,000/mm in the absence of drugs known to cause thrombocytopenia.
10. Immunologic disorder: Any of the following laboratory tests: positive LE cell preparation; Anti-DNA antibodies; Anti-Sm antibodies; false positive serologic latex test for syphilis which remains positive for at least 6 months along with a negative fluorescent treponemal antibody absorption (FTPA) test.
11. Antinuclear antibody (ANA): An abnormal ANA titer performed by immunofluorescent or equivalent assay methods at any time, and in the absence of drugs known to cause drug related lupus.

Diagnostic Criteria for Sjögren's Syndrome

For a diagnosis of Sjögren's syndrome, an autoimmune disorder typically characterized by sicca syndrome (oral and ocular dryness), three out of four of the following diagnostic criteria must be met: dry eyes (keratoconjunctivitis sicca), dry mouth, either a positive antibody test for SSA (Ro) or a positive minor salivary gland biopsy with a focus score of 1 or greater. However, exceptions are made for patients with hepatitis C or patients using medications known to alter salivary gland flow. For these individuals, only two symptoms are required for diagnosis.

Diagnostic Criteria for Inclusion Body Myositis

The autoimmune muscle disorder inclusion body myositis is diagnosed by a combination of clinical and laboratory features and family history. Clinical features include: illness occurring for more than 6 months, age of onset greater than 30 years old, muscle weakness affecting proximal and distal muscles of arms and legs, and either finger flexor weakness, wrist flexor weakness more pronounced than wrist extensor weakness, or quadriceps muscle weakness equal or less than grade 4.

Laboratory features include serum creatine kinase (CK) levels less than 12 times normal, muscle biopsy changes including mononuclear cell invasion of non-necrotic muscle fibers, vacuolated muscle fibers and either amyloid deposits or 15–18 nm tubulofilaments, and electromyography results consistent with inflammatory myopathy.

Rarely, inclusion body myositis is observed in families in a condition different from hereditary inclusion body myopathy, which is not associated with inflammation. Therefore, patients with inclusion body myositis must have a family history of documented inflammation.

When Diagnostic Criteria are Incomplete

Often, certain disorders seem likely, but the established diagnostic criteria can't be met. In this case, the diagnosis is one of "possible disease." Regarding inclusion body myositis, if the muscle biopsy shows inflammation and other laboratory and clinical features are present, but there is no evidence of the pathological changes needed for diagnosis, then a diagnosis of possible inclusion body myositis can be made.[1]

LABORATORY TESTS

Laboratory tests help diagnose which organs or bodily systems are affected. For instance, an abnormally low platelet count occurs in thrombocytopenia, a clotting disorder. Platelet antibody tests are used to determine if the patient has autoimmune or idiopathic thrombocytopenia rather than a drug induced disorder.

However, organ-specific and immunological changes may not be apparent early on. For instance, in the early stages of autoimmune liver disease, organ specific enzymes, such as alkaline phosphatase, an enzyme that typically reflects liver cell damage, may be normal. And titers for specific liver associated autoantibodies may be negative or low.

Compounding the problem, most autoantibodies aren't specific for one disease. While certain positive tests in an autoantibody panel might suggest an underlying AD, the results may point to several different disorders. And where tests for HLA antigens might be helpful, there is also a considerable overlap between diseases.

Antibody Panels

For most connective tissue, arthralgic, or autoimmune thyroid diseases, an antibody panel is used to aid in diagnosing the specific AD. In September of 2000, the RhiGene Autoantibody Screening Kit was introduced. Using one small blood sample, this kit simultaneously detects circulating antinuclear, antimitochondrial, parietal cell, smooth muscle and reticulin autoantibodies in an indirect immunofluorescent test system. Used as a semiquantitative (positive or negative results) determination, the test aids in the diagnosis of SLE, chronic autoimmune liver diseases, pernicious anemia and other related ADs.

Panels are sometimes use to help diagnose organ specific ADs. For example, if liver disease is present or suspected, patients are tested for a panel of different autoantibodies. Antimitochondrial antibodies (AMA) are present in nearly 100 percent of patients with primary biliary cirrhosis (PBC). Autoimmune cholangitis has the same symptoms as PBC, but patients do not have AMA or if they do, the titers are very low. Smooth muscle antibodies are present in autoimmune hepatitis but not in PBC.

Antinuclear Antibody Tests

Most patients suspected of having connective tissue disorders are tested for antinuclear antibodies (ANA). ANA, which include a number of different subtypes, target the nucleus of various cells located throughout the body. Thus, they're more often associated with systemic rather than organ specific disorders. However, ANA are commonly seen in patients with other ADs besides the rheumatic diseases, and they're occasionally seen in normal, healthy persons.

ANA are present in high titers in most connective tissue disorders such as systemic lupus erythematosus (SLE) and in 40 percent to 70 percent of patients with Sjögren's syndrome. The ANA test is also positive in 40 percent to 70 percent of patients with polymyositis and dermato-mysositis.[2]

ANA are also often present, although usually at lower concentrations or titers, in patients with Graves' disease, autoimmune hepatitis, Hashimoto's thyroiditis, and primary biliary cirrhosis. Despite these limitations, the ANA test can aid in diagnosing or ruling out certain specific disorders.

For instance, a patient who reports having symptoms of SLE can be expected to have a high (greater than 1:640) ANA titer if SLE is the cause. A negative titer in this patient suggests that an autoimmune connective tissue disorder is unlikely. A patient with Graves' disease who complains of joint pain and has a high ANA titer likely has a second AD, whereas patients with positive, but low ANA titers, probably do not have a concomitant disorder, although it's recommended that they be retested in several months.

ANA Test Interpretation

Interpretation of ANA test results involves identifying different appearances or patterns of immunofluorescent (IF) staining when patient serum is added to tissue from a humoral tumor cell line substrate known as the Hep-2 cell line. The pattern of the ANA, (speckled or rimmed) can also help identify which particular nuclear antigens, and, therefore, which rheumatic diseases, are likely to be present. When serum is reactive after being diluted 1:80, the test is considered positive.

Antibodies to the DNA-histone complex, also referred to as the nucleosome, are associated with SLE while double stranded (ds) DNA antibodies are seen in SLE but not in drug related lupus. The speckled pattern may be produced by antibodies to Smith (Sm), ribonucleoprotein (RNP), Ro (also known as SSA), La (also known as SSb), Scl-70, centromere, pericytoplasmic nuclear antigen (PCNA) and other antigens. Many of these antibodies, but not all, are associated with Sjögren's syndrome, mixed connective tissue disease, scleroderma, SLE, and rheumatoid arthritis.

When the speckled pattern occurs, patients should be tested for antibodies to specific members of this group in a test for extractable nuclear antigens (ENA). Moderate to high antibodies directed toward dsDNA or Sm are very specific for SLE, although dsDNA titers can fluctuate with disease activity. Antibodies to RNP are associated with mixed connective tissue disease (MCTD), an autoimmune disorder with symptoms overlapping those of SLE, inflammatory myositis and scleroderma. Antibodies to SSA and SSB are associated with Sjögren's syndrome.

Antibodies to centromere occur in patients with CREST syndrome, manifested by skin hardening over the fingers, Raynaud's phenomenon (blanching and numbness of fingers upon exposure to cold), esophageal problems, and calcium deposits over the fingertips. Scl-70 antibodies are associated with scleroderma, and anti-histone antibodies are associated with both SLE and drug related lupus.

Prognostic Applications

The ANA test is also helpful in providing information concerning prognosis. However, the prevalence of positive ANA results in patients with Raynaud phenomenon varies depending on the population studied. And while Raynaud phenomenon is often associated with several rheumatic diseases, including SLE, RA and scleroderma, up to 81 percent of patients with Raynaud phenomenon never go on to develop a systemic rheumatic disease. A positive ANA test in a patient with Raynaud phenomenon increases the likelihood of developing a systemic rheumatic disease from approximately 19 percent to 30 percent, while a negative ANA test result decreases the likelihood to about 7 percent.[3]

RF Factor

The test for rheumatoid factor (RF) test is often ordered at the same time as the ANA. RF is an antibody to a specific portion (Fc portion) of immunoglobulin G (IgG). Its origin is unknown, but it is found in most patients with rheumatoid arthritis (RA) and other rheumatic disorders. RFs are detected in up to 80 percent of adults with RA and often at high titers in repeated tests. However, RFs also occur in other connective tissue diseases, in chronic infectious diseases such as infective endocarditis, tuberculosis, and hepatitis B, and in lower titers in up to 20 percent of the normal elderly population.

Autoantibodies and Associated Diseases

A number of other specific autoantibody tests are often used to help diagnose ADs. Certain positive autoantibody tests also help predict systemic organ involvement. For instance, in addition to having inflammatory infiltration and muscle destruction, patients with dermatomyositis or polymyositis who have antibodies to aminoacyl-tRNA syntheases, including anti-Jo-1, are likely to have pulmonary involvement and arthritis.

Patients with scleroderma are classified into two distinct disease types, limited and diffuse or systemic. Patients with limited disease (also known as CREST syndrome) tend to have a better prognosis than those who have diffuse disease.

Autoantibodies can help distinguish the two disease types. Limited disease is associated with the anticentromere pattern of ANA staining. Diffuse disease is associated with autoantibodies to the enzyme DNA topoisomerase-1 (anti-Scl-70) or to components of nucleoli. Scleroderma patients with anti-Scl-70 autoantibodies tend to have more severe organ involvement, especially pulmonary fibrosis. [4]

Patients with mixed connective tissue disease (MCTD) pose a diagnostic challenge since their signs and symptoms are similar to those seen in SLE, scleroderma and myositis. A test for anti-nRNP autoantibodies is helpful in diagnosing MCTD since these autoantibodies are commonly seen in MCTD but not in the other disorders.

In patients with neuropathy, a condition that can occur as a complication of diabetes or tumors or as a primary AD, antibody tests are invaluable. Most patients with autoimmune idiopathic autonomic neuropathy have nicotinic acetylcholine receptor antibodies. Furthermore, levels of these antibodies typically decrease as patients favorably respond to treatment.[5] The following list describes specific autoantibody tests that are often used to help rule out or diagnose specific ADs.

Acetylcholine Receptor Antibodies—Primarily seen in autoimmune myasthenia gravis; positive results may occur in a small number of patients with Graves' disease and autoimmune liver disease and in 13 percent of patients with lupus.

Antineutrophil Cytoplasmic Autoantibodies (ANCA)—Primarily seen in necrotizing vasculitis involving many different tissues; very useful in the diagnosis of Wegener's granulomatosis (84 percent—100 percent of patients), microscopic polyarteritis, systemic vasculitis, and idiopathic necrotizing and crescentic glomerulonephritis; ANCA represent a family of autoantibodies with varied specificities against myeloid-specific protein;[6] subtypes of ANCA include:

   C-ANCA—Cytoplasmic staining ANCA that parallels disease activity in up to 85 percent of patients with Wegener's granulomatosis and vasculitis.

P-ANCA—Perinuclear staining ANCA primarily found in inflammatory bowel diseases (IBD), including Crohn's disease and ulcerative colitis (59 percent–84 percent of patients); present in up to 85 percent of patients with primary sclerosing cholangitis, both with and without IBD.

Atypical P-ANCA—Different types of P-ANCA are seen in IBD and in patients with liver disease. While the P-ANCA in IBD appear typical and resemble those seen in vasculitic diseases, the antibodies seen in primary sclerosing cholangitis (PSC) and autoimmune hepatitis are atypical. These antibodies appear to react with a protein in the nucleus, rather than the cytoplasm, of neutrophilic white blood cells.

Antiphospholipid Antibodies—includes lupus anticoagulant and cardiolipin antibodies. Cardiolipin antibodies and the lupus anticoagulant marker are often seen in lupus patients although, as with most antibodies, they tend to come and go, occurring more frequently in the active disease state. Antiphospholipid antibodies interfere with the normal function of blood vessels, by causing a narrowing and irregularity of the vessel and by causing abnormal clotting or thrombosis.

C1q Autoantibodies—primarily found in patients (nearly 100 percent) with complement deficiency associated urticarial vasculitis syndrome, and in 77 percent of patients with rheumatoid vasculitis and 71 percent of patients with systemic lupus erythematasus (SLE).

Cardiolipin (Phospholipid) Antibodies—Primarily seen in SLE, Antiphospholipid Syndrome (APS), connective tissue diseases and spontaneous thromboses. Anticardiolipin antibody is increased in pregnant women with lupus who have had miscarriages. The combination of thrombotic (clotting) problems, miscarriages, and a low platelet count is called the Antiphospholipid Syndrome. This syndrome may occur in women who do not have lupus. Patients who have had strokes or heart attacks at an early age or unexplained miscarriages should be tested for these antibodies.

Cathepsin G antibodies—Primarily seen in patients with SLE; these antibodies have recently been found in the immune complex deposits of glomerulonephritis.

Centromere antibodies—Primarily seen in patients with CREST syndrome.

Cytoplasmic Neutrophil Antibodies (ANCA, cANCA, which produces a different staining pattern)—ANCA are found in vasculitis including patients with anti–GBM mediated renal disease and lupus glomerulonephritis; cANCA are primarily seen in active Wegener's granulomatosis (WG).

DNA Antibodies—Native or double-stranded (ds) DNA is seen primarily in SLE. Levels of dsDNA > 20 U/ml are consistent with a diagnosis of SLE. Single stranded (ss) DNA antibodies are seen in patients with SLE and DRL. Low titers of ssDNA and dsDNA are occasionally seen in normal healthy individuals and in patients with other autoimmune disorders.

Endomysial Antibodies—Seen in 70 percent to 80 percent of patients with dermatitis herpetiformis or celiac disease and in nearly all such patients who have high grade GSE and are not adhering to a gluten free diet.

Erythrocyte Antibodies—Primarily seen in autoimmune hemolytic anemia.

Extractable Nuclear Antigen (ENA) Antibodies—Primarily seen in patients with connective tissue or rheumatic diseases; includes antibodies to SSA, SSb, Sm and RNP.

Fibrillarin Antibodies—Primarily seen in immune complex glomeru-loneprhritis triggered by mercuric chloride; antifibrillarin antibodies are also seen in a subset of scleroderma associated with elevated mercury levels.

Gliadin Antibodies—Primarily seen in GSE and dermatitis herpetiformis; tests should measure both IgG and IgM gliadin antibodies.

Ganglionic Acetylcholine Receptor Antibodies—Primarily seen in idiopathic autonomic neuropathy disorders, which, other than their autoimmune component, are clinically indistinguishable from the subacute autonomic neuropathy that may accompany lung cancer or other tumors; most often occur as autoantibodies to the nicotinic acetylcholine receptor.[7]

Glomerular Basement Membrane Antibodies (GBM)—Primarily seen in patients with untreated glomerulonephritis and/or pulmonary hemorrhage (Goodpasture's syndrome). Anti–GBM are the cause of disease in glomerulonephritis, Goodpasture's syndrome, and less commonly, idiopathic pulmonary hemosiderosis. The production of GBM is usually self-limited but these antibodies may mediate irreversible renal failure.

Glutamic Acid Decarboxylase Antibodies—Found in up to 60 percent of patients with Stiff Man Syndrome (SMS). Up to 1/3 of SMS patients with positive glutamic acid decarboxylase antibody titers also have IDDM.

Herpes Gestationis Autoantibodies—Primarily seen in patients with herpes gestationis (71 to 89 percent of patients) and bullous pemphigoid (47 percent to 53 percent of patients) disorders.

Histone Antibodies—Primarily seen in SLE and DRL; histone is the protein component of DNA.

Insulin Autoantibodies—Primarily seen in untreated patients with insulin dependent diabetes mellitus (IDDM). Insulin antibodies, however, include islet cell autoantibodies.

Intrinsic Factor Blocking Antibodies—Primarily seen in pernicious anemia (PA); these antibodies are more likely to be present in PA patients who are African-Americans or Latin-Americans than in white patients.

Islet Cell Autoantibodies (ICA)—Primarily seen in 80 percent of newly diagnosed IDDM patients. ICA are directed against the beta cells of the pancreatic islets.

Jo-1 Antibodies—Primarily seen in polymyositis.

Liver/Kidney Micrcrosome (LKM-1) Antibodies—Primarily in subtype 2 of chronic autoimmune hepatitis, a disorder that predominantly affects children.

Lupus anticoagulant—Type of circulating antibody associated with prolonged coagulation screening tests; seen in patients with lupus and antiphospholipid syndrome; highly associated with the presence of antiphospholipid antibodies.

Mitochondrial Antibodies—Seen in 79 percent to 94 percent of patients with primary biliary cirrhosis (PBC) and up to 25 percent of patients with Graves' disease.

Mitotic Spindle Apparatus Autoantibodies—Primarily seen in rheumatoid arthritis, Sjögren's syndrome, Hashimoto thyroiditis and localized scleroderma as well as respiratory infections, dilated cardiomyopathy and melanoma.

Myelin Basic Protein Antibodies—Primarily seen in the spinal fluid of patients with multiple sclerosis (77 percent of patients), optic neuritis, and experimental allergic encephalomyelitis. Myelin basic protein antibody titers are highly correlated to exacerbation and relapse in MS.

Myeloperoxidase Antibodies (aMPO)—Subset of ANCA which forms pANCA staining pattern in ANA tests; seen primarily in autoimmune vasculitis, usually in patients with renal involvement characterized by necrotizing glomerulonephritis; these antibodies have recently been found in the immune complex deposits of glomerulonephritis.

Myocardial Antibodies—Primarily seen in patients with acute rheumatic fever and carditis, in patients who have sustained mechanical (surgical or traumatic) or ischemic damage to myocardial tissue in the post cardiotomy and post myocardial infarction syndromes.

Neurofilament Heavy Subunit Autoantibodies—Primarily seen in neurodegenerative disorders including neuropsychiatric SLE, thymic tumors associated with myasthenia gravis (MG), and spongiform encephalopathies.

Neuronal Autoantibodies—Primarily seen in neuropsychiatric SLE, where positive titers are seen in up to 75 percent of patients; also seen in antiphospholipid syndrome and Raynaud's phenomenon.

Nucleolar Antibodies—The most widely recognized nucleolar antibodies include anti-Pm-Scl, anti-RNA polymerase I-III, anti-U3-RNP (antifibrillarin) and anti-Th (To RNP). The Anti-nucleolar antibodies are fairly specific for scleroderma. Anti-Pm-Scl is most often associated with inflammatory myopathy in conjunction with scleroderma, whereas anti-U3-RNP is most often seen in African-Americans with scleroderma, especially those with more severe diffuse disease. Anti-RNA polymerase I has also been associated with rapidly progressive diffuse scleroderma, with a high prevalence of internal organ involvement. In contrast, anti-Th To antibodies are usually seen in limited skin disease. Antinucleolar antibodies may also occur in patients with SLE, Sjögren's syndrome, rheumatoid arthiritis, and Raynaud's phenomenon.

Polymer Antibodies—Primarily seen in women with silicone breast implants exhibiting moderate to severe symptoms of autoimmune disease.

Rheumatoid Factors (RF)—Autoantibodies reactive with the crystallizable fragment (Fc fragment) of immunoglobulin G (IgG); found in 50 percent to 90 percent of patients with rheumatoid arthritis with higher levels in active disease that correlate inversely with functional capacity. Also seen in 75 percent to 95 percent of SS patients, 50 percent to 60 percent of patients with MCTD, 25 percent to 40 percent of patients with IgA nephropathy, 15 percent to 35 percent of patients with SLE, 20 percent to 30 percent of patients with systemic sclerosis and a variable percent of patients with cryoglobulinemia.

Ribonuclear Protein (RNP, U1 RNP) Antibodies—Primarily seen in mixed connective tissue disease (MCTD) and SLE (35 percent to 45 percent of patients); patients with SLE or MCTD who only have RNP antibodies have a decreased prevalence of renal diseases and generally favorable prognosis.[8]

Ribosomal P Protein (RPP) Autoantibodies—Primarily seen in patients with SLE who have related conditions of severe depression or psychosis; however, a positive test is not diagnostic for lupus psychosis because almost

50 percent of patients with RPP do not have severe behavioral problems.[9] RPP are also seen in 7 percent to 20 percent of patients with SLE. RRP are also occasionally found in Sjögren's syndrome associated with SLE and central nervous system involvement. RRP are also seen in all patients with lupus hepatitis.

Scl 70 Antibodies—Primarily seen in scleroderma and in sclerosing cholangitis.

Silicate Autoantibodies—Primarily seen in patients with breast implants, vascular prostheses, and joint repair and replacement. Their diagnostic significance is unclear although a relationship to fibromyalgia has recently been suggested.

Skin Autoantibodies—Primarily seen in bullous skin diseases.

Smith (Sm) Antibodies—Primarily seen in SLE, where it occurs in most patients who fit the diagnostic criteria for SLE.

Smooth Muscle Antibodies (SMA)—Primarily seen in chronic autoimmune hepatitis and in patients with active hepatitis caused by toxins such as alcohol.

SSA (Ro) Antibodies—Primarily seen in Sjögren's syndrome and SLE.

SSB (La) Antibodies—Primarily seen in Sjögren's syndrome and SLE.

Striational Autoantibodies—Primarily occur in patients with MG who have thymoma; also found in 55 percent of older MG patients but rarely in patients who are less than 20 years old.

Thyroglobulin Antibodies (ATG)—Primarily seen in Hashimoto's thyroiditis (HT); also seen to a lesser extent in Graves' disease and other autoimmune thyroid disorders.

Thyroid Peroxidase (TPO) Antibodies—Primarily seen in HT and to a lesser extent in Graves' disease and other autoimmune thyroid disorders.

Thyrotropin (TSH) Receptor Antibodies (TRAb)—Stimulating TRAb are seen in Graves' disease; binding TRAb are seen in all forms of autoimmune thyroid disease; blocking TRAb are seen in HT and primary myxedema and are associated with Graves' Ophthalmopathy.

Tubulin Autoantibodies—Primarily seen in severe neurological diseases, including chronic inflammatory demyelinating polyradiculoneuropathy (CIPD), Guillain-Barré syndrome, diabetic neuropathy and SLE. High titers of tubulin autoantibodies are also seen in the serum and spinal fluid of patients with MS, Alzheimer's disease, optic neuritis and amyotrophic lateral sclerosis (ALS).[10]

Voltage-Gated Calcium Channel Autoantibodies—Primarily seen in Lambert-Easton myasthenic syndrome (LEMS), an autoimmune disease associated with small-cell lung cancer; in LEMS, 4 different subtypes of these autoantibodies target voltage-gated calcium channels situated on the presynaptic nerve, impairing neurotransmitter release from the neuromuscular junction.

Miscellaneous Laboratory Tests

Laboratory tests that indicate inflammation are also helpful. The following list represents some of the miscellaneous tests used to help diagnose autoimmune disorders.

C-Reactive Protein (CRP)

C-reactive protein (pentraxin) is typically elevated in acute phase response to infections, tissue damage and inflammation. Levels of CRP often rise 100 to 1,000 fold within 24 hours of an inflammatory attack or infection. However, in collagen diseases, including SLE, CRP concentrations are usually normal.

In rheumatoid arthritis, persistently elevated CRP levels (>4 mg/dl) are present during the active disease state, although levels fall during periods of remission. CRP is also elevated in chronically active HLA B27 positive incidences of ankylosing spondylitis. CRP is also elevated in appendicitis, strokes and heart attacks.

Cytokine and Complement Tests

A number of autoimmune diseases are associated with changes in cytokine and complement levels. For instance, patients with SLE are typically deficient in total complement, particularly the C3 and C4 fractions. Complement functions in a series of steps known as a cascade, in which various complement components are activated.

Complement, like antibodies, are proteins found in serum, the liquid portion of blood. However, while antibodies target and lock on to specific antigens, complement proteins attack any particle lacking the "self" marker. Since complement change over time, and their levels are indicative of disease severity, measurements of C3 and C4 are often used to diagnose the active disease state in patients with SLE.

Immune complexes of complement and antibody may also be measured in a test known as the C1Q binding assay for immune complexes. Immune complexes typically cause deposits, which are associated with glomerulonephritis and arthritic syndromes.

Outside of research, cytokine levels are not presently measured in the United States. However, they are markers of inflammation and a number of different autoimmune diseases are associated with elevated or decreased levels of specific cytokines. For instance, in some experimental studies, interleukin-1beta (IL-1β) measurements are found to correlate with disease activity and pain scores.

C1Q Complement Component

C1 is composed of C1q, C1r, and C1s. C1q recognizes and binds to immunoglobulin (autoantibody) molecules that are complexed to antigen. Upon recognizing these immune complexes, C1q initiates the complement cascade. This test is used to differentiate congenital complement deficiency states from acquired conditions such as SLE.

Total Complement CH 50 or CH 100

The complement system consists of at least 15 plasma proteins that interact sequentially in a cascade effect. The end result can be cell lysis or destruction, release of histamine from mast cells and platelets, increased vascular permeability, contraction of smooth muscles, changes to leukocytes and neutralization of certain viruses.

The CH 50 and CH 100 assays measure complement by assessing the amount of serum required to lyse 50 percent and 100 percent, respectively, of indicator testing cells. Decreased levels are found in infectious and autoimmune diseases associated with complement fixation and consumption. Low levels are indicative of exacerbations or flares in patients with SLE or glomerulonephritis.

C3

The classic and alternative complement pathways converge at the third or C3 step of the complement cascade. Most diseases with immune complex activity show decreased C3 levels. C3 levels are decreased in malnutrition, liver disease, immune complex disease, SLE, SS, RA, paroxysmal nocturnal hemoglobinuria, autoimmune hemolytic anemia, and in 75 percent of patients with membrane proliferative glomerulonephritis.

C3 is increased in acute phase of rheumatic diseases, including RA and SLE, as well as acute viral hepatitis, myocardial infarction, cancer, diabetes, pregnancy, sarcoidiosis and thyroiditis.

C4

Another member of the complement cascade, C4 is decreased in SLE, RA, proliferative glomerulonephritis, hereditary angiodema and decreased protein states such as burns. C4 is increased in various malignancies and is not considered clinically useful.

Cold Agglutinins

This test is positive in patients with cold agglutinin syndrome. In this syndrome, cold agglutinins, usually IgM with antibodies to I antigen, attach to the patient's red blood cells causing a variety of symptoms, including chronic hemolytic anemia.

Cyroglobulin

An abnormal protein seen in some autoimmune disorders, cryoglobulins have three subtypes: type I or monoclonal, type II or mixed, and type III or polyclonal. Type I cryoglobulins are associated with monoclonal macroglobulinemia or multiple myeloma. The presence of type II cryoglobulins is associated with essential mixed cryoglobulinemia, vasculitis, glomeruloneprhritis, SLE, RA and Sjögren's syndrome.

Direct Coombs Test

The direct coombs test detects antibodies that are bound to the surface of circulating red blood cells (erythrocytes). The test is positive in autoimmune hemolytic anemia although many different drugs can also cause a positive direct coombs test.

Erythrocyte Sedimentation Rate (ESR, Sed Rate)

The erythrocyte sedimentation test measures the rate in which red cells settle when placed in a vertical test tube. The sedimentation rate is directly proportional to the weight of the cell aggregate and inversely proportional to the surface area. The ESR is markedly elevated in blood protein disorders and in inflammatory disorders. Moderate elevations are commonly seen in active inflammatory diseases, including rheumatoid arthritis, collagen diseases, and chronic infections.

HLA B27

HLA B27 is one of the human leukocyte antigens found as a marker on lymphocytes. Up to 89 percent of white patients with ankylosing spondylitis are positive for HLA B27, and about 50 percent of black patients are positive for HLA B27. The HLA B27 antgen is also present in 42 percent of individuals with juvenile rheumatoid arthritis and 79 percent of individuals with Reiter's syndrome. Approximately 8 percent of the normal population may carry the HLA B27 antigen. Thus, this test is not diagnostic for ankylosing spondylitis, rheumatoid arthritis or Reiter's syndrome without other collaborating data.

SR Proteins

Researchers at Fred Hutchinson Cancer Research Center have identified a group of proteins known as SR proteins that appear in the blood of patients with lupus. This test is said to be positive in up to 70 percent of lupus patients.

Lumbar Puncture (LP)

A lumbar puncture (LP) or spinal tap is performed in order to obtain cerebrospinal fluid (CSF) for analysis. LP involves inserting a hollow needle with a stylus into the lumbar region of the spinal canal. CSF is tested for cells, protein and glucose abnormalities, and infectious agents. Spinal fluid may also be tested for the presence of autoantibodies and certain abnormal proteins. Oligoclonal IgM bands, for instance, are seen in 28 percent of patients with MS. Furthermore, in neuro–Behçet disease, oligoclonal IgM and IgA bands are detected mainly in the active stages of the disease. In one study, eighty-one percent of patients with progressive neuro– Behçet's disease had a CSF IgM Index >0.070 and showed a marked increase in interleukin-6 (IL-6) activity.[11]

The MRZ reaction is also useful in diagnosing MS. The MRZ reaction reflects increased antibody indices to measles, rubella and varicella zoster. If assays for oligoclonal immunoglobulins are combined with the MRZ reaction, abnormal results are obtained in 99 percent of patients with MS. Furthermore, the presence of anti-carbohydrate binding protein (lectin) antibodies in the CSF of MS patients younger than 50 is a specific test, with 96 percent of patients with clinically definite MS and 95 percent positive of those with probable MS being positive.[12]

Myelin basic protein antibodies are also commonly found in the CSF of patients with MS. Both cellular and humoral immune responses are involved in the inflammatory demyelination seen in MS. Therefore, this test is useful in detecting disease activity in both MS and in virus-induced demyelination syndromes.

ACTH Stimulation Test

In this test, blood or urine cortisol levels are measured before and after a synthetic form of adrenocorticotrophin hormone (ACTH) is administered by injection. Normally, this will cause a rise in cortisol levels. In Addison's disease and other disorders of adrenal insufficiency, the cortisol level shows little or no change after ACTH administration.

Urinalysis

A routine urine exam is useful in detecting certain abnormalities or complications such as kidney disease, glucose intolerance, liver disease, and infection.

IMAGING TESTS

Imaging tests are frequently used to assess changes in the muscles or brain that are characteristic of certain autoimmune diseases.

Skull Films

Skull films generally include anteroposterior and lateral radiographic views although other angles may be included. Skull films demonstrate skull fracture, pressure changes indicated by displacement of the pineal gland, unusual calcification, the size and shape of skull bones, bone erosion and abnormal vascularity. Skull films are useful in ruling out head trauma and tumor as a cause of neurological symptoms.

Chest X-Rays

Chest x-rays are often used to diagnose pulmonary or cardiac abnormalities, including inflammation.

Computed Axial Tomography (CAT) Scan

Computed axial tomography was first introduced in England in 1972. In this procedure, which sometimes uses contrast dye, the patient lies flat on a table, and a movable circular frame encircles the head, revolving around it while taking radiographic readings. Denser structures such as bone can be differentiated from less dense areas such as cerebrospinal fluid. On CAT scans, areas of the brain can be differentiated into spinal fluid, blood, white or gray matter, congealed blood, bone or calcification. CAT scans can differentiate multiple sclerosis from conditions caused by tumors and strokes.

Magnetic Resonance Imaging (MRI)

Magnetic resonance images of the body's hydrogen distribution are useful in differentiating tissue constituents, such as the gray and white matter of the brain. More than 90 percent of MS patients have abnormal scans with darkened areas indicating tissue destruction. In particular, the blood-brain barrier shows inflammation using MRI. Damage to this tissue allows some harmful substances to pass into the brain. The dissolution of the blood-brain barrier is considered the first step in the development of the characteristic lesions seen in MS.

MRI is particularly effective in detecting necrotic tissue, oxygen-deprived tissue, small malignancies and degenerative diseases within the central nervous system. MRI can identify cerebral and spinal cord edema, hemorrhage, vascular malformations, tumors of the brain and brain stem, and congenital abnormalities.

Ultrasonography

Ultrasonography is based on the principle that the body's tissues have a property called acoustic impedance, or ability to react with sound waves. Sound waves that enter tissue can be transmitted through tissue or reflected. Cystic or calcified tissue will react differently than normal tissue. Using a technique called Doppler imaging, the vascular system of tissue can also be examined, making it an essential tool for the study of deep vein thrombosis associated with antiphospholipid syndrome. Ultrasound is useful in determining glandular changes, such as the salivary gland changes seen in patients with Sjögren's syndrome.

Positron Emission Transaxial Tomography (PETT) Scan

Unlike CAT or MRI, which look at anatomy or body structure, PETT provides information on body chemistry and cell function. The patient is first injected with a radioactive sugar called fluorodeoxyglucose (FDG). Certain cells, including cancer cells, metabolize glucose faster. As the radioactive compound is distributed throughout the body, the PETT scanner detects areas that are using higher than normal amounts of sugar.

BIOLOGICAL RECORDINGS

Electroencephalogram

The electroencephalogram (EEG) is a recording of the electrical activity of the brain (brain waves). Surface electrodes are attached to scalp to record the electrical signals from the brain, which are interpreted as different rhythms. An EEG is particularly useful for differentiating functional from organic brain syndromes. Conventional EEG is abnormal in 70 percent to 80 percent of patients with neuropsychiatric SLE. The EEG is also useful in revealing unsuspected seizure activity in autoimmune disease patients.

Echoencephalogram

An encephalogram (ECHO) is a simple test that uses pulsating ultrasonic waves to indicate deviation of the midline structures. A probe is place on the midaxis, which corresponds to the temporal bones of the skull. The probe contains a transducer and emits an ultrasonic beam that travels through the patient's skull. The reflected waves are recorded and are useful in detecting changes in the brain such as space-occupying lesions. Often, brain lesions must be ruled out to diagnose autoimmune neurological disorders.

Electromyography

Electromyography (EMG) is used to record the electrical activity of muscle and its peripheral nerves. EMG is used to detect the presence and type of neuromuscular disorders that affect the lower motor neuron, the neuromuscular junctions, skeletal muscle fibers, the primary sensory neuron, and the voluntary and reflex activity of muscles. The EMG can detect minimal nerve impairment in an isolated muscle.

The procedure involves insertion of needle electrodes into the muscle to be examined. Although the procedure is not painful, an uncomfortable sensation is usually felt. Recordings are made of the electrical activity of the muscle at rest and during contraction. Normally, there is no electrical activity of a muscle at rest, whereas during voluntary contraction, the action potential is elevated. In lower motor nerve disease, fibrillations are observed. In muscle disease, decreased amplitude and duration are observed during muscle contraction.

Nerve Conduction Times

Nerve conduction times include measurements of the speed of the conduction of motor and sensory fibers in peripheral nerves. The motor conduction rate is measured by comparing the compound action potential caused by both distal and proximal stimulation during the latent period. Lowered values are found in neuropathy.

PATHOLOGY STUDIES

Biopsies

Biopsies are considered the gold standard for diagnosing several ADs, including Sjögren's syndrome (lip biopsy), primary biliary cirrhosis (liver biopsy) and celiac disease (intestinal biopsy). In SLE, kidney biopsies are used to determine the extent of immune complex mediated damage. In biopsies, a small amount of tissue is removed and examined for cellular changes characteristic of certain disease states. Biopsies may be performed during surgery, although today many biopsies are performed by alternate means, notably fine needle aspiration, with or without radiological guidance.

Fine Needle Aspiration

A number of needles, including suction needles and cutting needles, are available for fine needle aspiration (FNA). In FNA, which may be guided by imaging methods, a needle is inserted beneath the skin to a depth sufficient to obtain a tissue sample of the appropriate organ. The tissue sample is then examined by pathologists.

FNA is associated with a number of complications, including infection. The risk of adverse reactions is higher in certain procedures such as liver biopsy. The most ominous complication in liver biopsy is bleeding, which may occur in 0.005 percent to 0.3 percent of all biopsies. Bleeding may result from a tear in the capsule, laceration of the liver or development of fistula between a branch of the hepatic artery, portal vein and peritoneal cavity. Other complications include pneumothorax, perforation of the gallbladder, peritonitis, perforation of the duodenum and inadvertent renal biopsy.[13]

MISCELLANEOUS TESTS
FOR SPECIFIC DISORDERS

Neuropsychological Testing

Neuropsychological testing or assessment includes the evaluation of a wide range of cognitive, adaptive and emotional behaviors that reflect the function of the brain cortex. Testing is conducted by a clinical neuropsychologist over a period of 8 to 10 hours and is used to diagnose the absence or presence of an organic brain lesion.

Sialometry

Sialometry refers to the measurement of salivary gland flow. The procedure may be performed with or without stimulation using lemon juice. Both salivary and parotid gland flow are typically decreased in patients with Sjögren's syndrome. In salivary scintigraphy, radioactive material is injected into the gland, and gland function is measured by imaging tests. In sialography, dye is injected into the salivary gland, and an x-ray of the salivary duct system is taken.

Parotid Gland Flow

Parotid gland flow can be measured by applying a lashley cannula over the duct of the parotid gland with gentle suction. Flow from the submandibular gland is measured by using a tiny suction tip for a period of one minute.

Schirmer Test

The Schirmer test is used to measure lacrimal gland flow or tearing. In this test, small pieces of filter paper are placed between the lower eyelid and eyeball. The amount of wetting in 5 minutes is a rough indicator of tear production.

Rose Bengal and Lissamine Green Tests

These dyes are used to observe abnormal cells present on the surface of the eye.

Slit-lamp Exam

This test provides an indication of tear volume by magnifying the eye and viewing it in its resting state.

Radioiodine Uptake Test

The radioiodine uptake (RAI-U) test is used to measure the amount of iodine taken up by the thyroid gland. The patient drinks an oral suspension of radioactive iodine. Hours later, an imaging test is taken. Hyperthyroidism causes the thyroid to take up increased amounts of iodine, whereas in hypothyroidism decreased amounts are absorbed. The thyroid can also be scanned to see if nodules are present. RAI-U is not as specific as thyroid autoantibody tests for diagnosing autoimmune thyroid disorders.

7

The Autoimmune Disease Spectrum

Autoimmune diseases are classified according to the major organ or bodily system they affect, a tradition that developed in parallel with the specialization of medicine. It was thought that an endocrinologist, for example, would be best able to treat patients with Addison's disease. However, this approach doesn't address the underlying immune system defect in ADs. Furthermore, many ADs affect multiple organs.

For instance, patients with Sjögren's syndrome (SS) have oral and ocular dryness caused by autoimmune destruction of the glands that lubricate these organs. However, patients with SS may experience systemic glandular destruction of other mucous glands, including those in the vagina and stomach. Alternately, patients may have connective tissue involvement with full-blown rheumatological symptoms. Consequently, SS is considered a rheumatological disorder. Patients diagnosed with SS are generally referred to rheumatologists although they may only have symptoms of oral dryness.

This chapter discusses the etiology, immune system characteristics, and treatment applications for AD prototypes. The following list represents the major classifications of AD with examples of the type of disorders included in each category.

CLASSIFICATIONS OF AUTOIMMUNE DISEASE

Rheumatological Conditions

Includes disorders that affect the joints, connective tissue, and collagen: ankylosing spondylitis; CREST syndrome (seen in connective tissue diseases, including: scleroderma and dermatomyositis C = calcinosis cutis; R = Raynaud's phenomenon; E = esophageal dysmotility; S = scleroderma; T = telangiectasias), juvenile rheumatoid arthritis; mixed connective tissue disease (MCTD); peyronie's syndrome; polymyalgia rheumatica; Reiter's disease; rheumatoid arthritis (RA); scleroderma; Sjögren's syndrome; and systemic lupus erythematosus (SLE).

Muscle Disorders

Includes disorders that primarily affect muscle: cardiomyopathies; dermatomyositis; idiopathic inflammatory myopathies; myositis; polymyositis; and postmyocardial infarction syndrome.

Neurological Conditions

Includes disorders in which the nerve-muscle connection is impaired: chronic inflammatory demyelinating polyneuropathy (CIPD); myasthenia gravis (MG); multiple sclerosis (MS); and neurolopsychiatric systemic lupus erythematosus.

Endocrine Disorders

Includes disorders that affect the endocrine glands or their hormone production: Addison's disease; Graves' disease (GD); Hashimoto's thyroiditis (HT); Hashitoxicosis; insulin dependent diabetes mellitus (IDDM); polyglandular endocrine disorders, types I and II; and primary myxedema.

Gastrointestinal/Biliary Diseases

Includes disorders of the gastrointestinal tract and the liver: chronic active hepatitis (CAH) type 1 and 2; Crohn's disease; dermatitis herpetiforminns; gluten sensitivity enteropathy (GSE) or celiac disease; inflammatory bowel disease (IBS); pernicious anemia (PA); primary biliary cirrhosis (PBC); primary sclerosing cholangitis.

Nephrological Conditions

Includes disorders of the kidney: Goodpasture's disease; interstitial cystitis; and Wegener's granulomatosis.

Hematological Disorders

Includes disorders of the blood and its components: antiphospholipid syndrome (APS); autoimmune hemolytic anemia; autoimmune neutropenia; cryoglobulinemia; idiopathic thrombocytopenic purpura (ITP); and pernicious anemia.

Dermatological Diseases

Includes diseases that affect the dermal layers of the skin: alopecia areata; pemphigoid disorders; porphyria; psoriasis; and vitiligo.

Vascular Disorders

Disorders of the blood vessels and valves of the circulatory system: atherosclerosis; rheumatic fever; and vasculitis.

Reproductive System Disorders

Disorders affecting the reproductive organs and fertility: endometriosis; herpes gestationis; oophritis; orchitis; and sperm and testicular autoimmunity.

Ophthalmological Disorders

Disorders affecting the eye: Graves' ophthalmopathy; ocular cicatricial pemphigoid; sympathetic ophthalmia; and uveitis.

Autoimmune Ear Disorders

Immune-mediated disorders affecting the ear and its nerves: Meniere's disease and sensorineural hearing loss.

Chronic Inflammatory Disorders

Disorders causing chronic inflammation in one or more organs: Allergic rhinitis and Guillain-Barré syndrome.

Rare Disorders

Disorders with variable symptoms that affect small numbers of the population: autoimmune hyperlipidemia; Behçet's disease; Chagas' disease; Cogan's syndrome; and Dressler's syndrome.

THE AUTOIMMUNE DISEASE PROCESS

The primary disease process in ADs appears to be initiated by a combination of autoantibodies, immune complexes, immune system cells, complement, and cytokines. It's thought that environmental agents cause an initial inflammatory process, followed by a specific immune attack in which immune system cells recognize sensitized self-antigens and initiates an autoimmune response.

LIST OF AUTOIMMUNE DISEASES
COMPILED BY AARDA

- Lupus
- Crohn's disease
- Cardiomyopathy
- Hemolytic anemia
- Fibromyalgia*
- Insulin dependent diabetes

- Osteoarthritis
- Chaga's disease
- Uveitis
- Chronic inflammatory demyelinating polyneuropathy (CIDP)

- Graves' disease
- Ulcerative colitis
- Vasculitis
- Multiple sclerosis
- Myasthenia gravis
- Myositis
- Neutropenia
- Psoriasis
- Chronic fatigue syndrome*
- Juvenile arthritis
- Juvenile diabetes
- Scleroderma
- Psoriatic arthritis
- Raynaud's phenomenon
- Sjögren's syndrome
- Rheumatic fever
- Rheumatoid arthritis
- Sarcoidosis
- Idiopathic thrombocytopenic purpura (ITP)
- Hashimoto's disease
- Mixed connective tissue disease
- Herpes gestationis
- Interstitial cystitis
- Pernicious anemia
- Acute necrotizing hemorrhagic leukoencephalitis
- Alopecia areata
- Ankylosing spondylitis
- Primary biliary cirrhosis
- Anti–GBM nephritis
- Anti–TBM nephritis
- Antiphospholipid syndrome (APS)
- Polymyalgia rheumatica
- Polymyositis
- Autoimmune Addison's disease
- Chronic active hepatitis (Vitiligo)
- Autoimmune hyperlipidemia
- Autoimmune myocarditis
- Temporal arteritis
- Cicatricial pemphigoid/benign mucosal pemphigoid
- Cogan's syndrome
- Congenital heart block
- Coxsackie myocarditis
- Demyelinating neuropathies
- Dermatomyositis
- Discoid lupus
- Phacoantigenic uveitis
- Polyarteritis nodosa
- Dressler's syndrome
- Essential mixed cryoglobulinemia
- Evan's syndrome
- Experimental allergic encephalomyelitis (EAE)
- Goodpasture's syndrome
- Allergic rhinitis
- Guillain-Barré syndrome
- Hypogammaglobulinemia
- Inclusion body myositis
- Vesiculobullous dermatosis
- Wegener's granulomatosis
- Meniere's disease
- Immunoregulatory lipoproteins
- Lambert-Eaton syndrome
- Mooren's ulcer
- Celiac sprue
- Ocular cicatricial pemphigoid
- Pemhigus vulgaris
- Perivenous encephalomyelitis
- Postmyocardial infarction syndrome
- Postpericardiotomy syndrome
- Scleritis
- Sperm & testicular autoimmunity
- Stiff man syndrome
- Subacute bacterial endocarditis (SBE)
- Sympathetic ophthalmia
- Transverse myelitis & necrotizing myelopathy

List of Autoimmune Diseases (continued)

- Autoimmune thyroid disease
- Axonal & neuronal neuropathies
- Behçet's disease
- Bullous pemphigoid
- Allergic asthma

- Type 1 autoimmune
  polyglandular syndrome
- Type II autoimmune
  polyglandular syndrome
- (Endometriosis

*These diseases have not yet been officially classified as autoimmune but are strongly suspected to be related.

Adapted with permission of the American Autoimmune Related Diseases Association (AARDA), East Detroit Michigan, 2000.

This list is not inclusive. Some disorders, such as the neuropathies, vasculitides and dermatological disorders, including porphyria, have subtypes or variations. Also, in several references, atherosclerosis, lymphoma, amyotrophic lateral sclerosis (ALS) and schizophrenia are included because of their evident autoimmune pathology.

For instance, patients with schizophrenia show several different immunologic abnormalities including an increased prevalence of ANA and platelet antibodies, altered cytokine production and increased levels of soluble cytokine receptors. Still other diseases, including many inner ear diseases, are currently being studied to determine if they have an autoimmune origin. Currently, they are considered immune-mediated.

AUTOIMMUNE DISEASE MODELS

The follow section describes the disease mechanism for the most prevalent ADs. These mechanisms offer insight into other related conditions. For instance, many of the rare connective tissue and other systemic disorders have similar disease mechanisms to those seen in lupus and rheumatoid arthritis.

LUPUS DISORDERS

The four types of lupus disorders include: (1) discoid lupus erythematosus (DLE or cutaneous lupus), which primarily affects the skin when exposed to sunlight; (2) systemic lupus erythematosus (SLE), a systemic disorder which affects the skin as well as vital organs; (3) transient or neonatal lupus, which affects newborns temporarily when maternal antibodies cross the placental membrane; (4) drug related lupus (DRL), a disorder resembling SLE which is induced by more than 70 different medications. Individuals with DRL rarely have rheumatological symptoms, and the disorder generally resolves after the responsible drug is discontinued.

Systemic Lupus Erythematosus

Systemic lupus erythematosus (SLE), the most serious of the lupus disorders, is characterized by specific autoantibodies, a wide range of symptoms and diverse organ involvement. SLE has the propensity to damage every organ system, although it seems to have partiality for connective tissue in the joints, muscles and skin, and the membranes surrounding the lungs, heart, kidneys and brain. SLE can also affect the orbit or eye socket, the eyelid, the optic nerve and the blood vessels that supply the retina.

Symptoms include rashes (discoid and malar), mouth ulcers, hair loss, joint pain and swelling, low-grade fever, fatigue, kidney disease, pleurisy, pericarditis (inflammation of the heart's lining), arthralgia, hives, nausea, persistent headache, weight loss, vasculitis, anemia, intestinal pseudo-obstruction, sensory neuropathies, pulmonary abnormalities including cough and pulmonary hypertension, Raynaud phenomenon, hemolytic anemia, and nerve abnormalities.

The most common and most debilitating symptom is fatigue, although the initial complaint in most patients is joint pain, arthralgia. Tenderness, edema and effusions commonly accompany polyarthritis that is called symmetric (involving both sides of the body equally), nonerosive, and nondeforming. Heart murmurs may be present in up to 70 percent of patients. The criteria for establishing a diagnosis of lupus can be found in chapter six.

Skin lesions involving the face, trunk and extremities are common findings in SLE. These lesions take many forms, including the classic "butterfly" rash distributed over the cheeks and base of the nose, urticaria, maculopapular lesions, ulceration, and alopecia. The basal layer of the epidermis may exhibit degenerative and fibrinoid changes at the epidermal-dermal junction, which may be accompanied by immunoglobulin and complement deposits. SLE can be differentiated from other connective tissue diseases by these deposits. In scleroderma, dermatomyositis and chronic discoid lupus, deposits only appear in skin lesions.

Fibrinous pleuritis and pericarditis (inflammatory disorders of the chest cavity and around the heart) may occur in SLE and may cause fibrous thickening and partial or complete obliteration of serosal cavities. Furthermore, a nonbacterial form of endocarditis involving mitral and tricuspid valves is characteristic of SLE.

Incidence and Epidemiology

SLE occurs 5 to 9 times more frequently in women than men and primarily affects adults. However, men are more likely than women to develop both discoid lupus and drug related lupus. SLE is said to have a prevalence of 50.8 per 100,000 individuals. The nonwhite population is more likely to be affected.

Men with SLE generally experience different organ involvement from what is usually seen in women. Men are more likely to develop autoimmune hemolytic anemia and seizure disorders, and they are less likely to develop Sjögren's syndrome and alopecia. Men are also more likely to have low levels of the immune system protein C3 and high levels of lupus anticoagulant. Because of the protective effects of testosterone, men usually have less frequent flare-ups than women.

However, men are more likely to develop pulmonary fibrosis (scarring of lung tissue), hypertension, glaucoma and renal insufficiency (loss of kidney function). Because they are more likely to have high levels of lupus anticoagulant, men are also more likely to develop blood clots and myocardial infarctions.[1]

Environmental Triggers of SLE

Environmental triggers include exposure to ultraviolet radiation, infection, diet, therapeutic drugs, physical and mental stress and estrogens. The etiology of SLE is only partly understood, but the hallmark is an inappropriate immune response to several autoantigens, including native DNA, chromatin, nucleoproteins, nucleosomes, histones, phospholipids, myeloperoxidase, thyroglobulin and many other cellular components. The autoimmune response in SLE appears to be driven by several specific autoantigen responses, each under separate genetic control.

The Disease Mechanism in SLE

Autoantibodies, circulating immune complexes, T lymphocytes and cytokines all contribute to the pathology of SLE. The presence of multiple autoantibodies, decreased suppressor T lymphocytes, spontaneous B cell activation and impaired macrophage activity suggest that basic immune system defects lead to the loss of tolerance in SLE.

Contributory factors include genetic, hormonal and environmental influences. Genetic influences are suggested by the family clustering seen in SLE and the association with HLA DR 2 and HLA DR 3 antigens, as well as inherited complement deficiencies. Many studies implicate estrogen as a causative factor in the development of SLE , whereas androgens such as testosterone decrease the incidence of SLE.

Environmental factors are indicated by the DRL syndromes (see chapter 5) and by the fact that sunlight exposure is known to induce the development of SLE, and flare-ups of SLE are triggered by infections, hormonal fluctuations and exposure to ultraviolet radiation. Exposure to silica dust is also suspected of causing flare-ups.[2] However, other factors that modulate immune responses such as diet and stress must also be considered.

Autoantibodies in SLE

Several different types of autoantibodies are known to occur in SLE. Antibodies to the complement molecule C1q bind with C1q, reducing complement stores. Consequently, patients with SLE are deficient in complement. This reduces their resistance to infections, and puts them at risk for developing more autoantibodies.

Individuals who are genetically deficient in complement almost always develop a form of lupus, although most patients with SLE do not have a genetic complement deficiency. Autoantibodies to nuclear cell antigens (antinuclear antibodies or ANA) are positive in the active phases of SLE. By reacting with the cell nucleus, ANA are able to damage the cell when it's dividing or involved in protein synthesis.

Antibodies to DNA are involved in the pathogenesis of immune complex deposition and inflammation, particularly the nephritis (kidney inflammation), serositis (inflammation of the serous membranes resulting in pleuritis and pericarditis), and vasculitis typically seen in SLE. In active SLE, vasculitis with subendothelial fibrin deposits may involve small arteries, arterioles and capillaries of affected organs (kidneys, spleen, heart, lungs) and, rarely in the severest cases, acute necrotizing vasculitis may involve the entire vessel wall. In later stages, the tissue surrounding blood vessels becomes fibrotic or scarred. The small arteries of the spleen typically develop concentric laminations near their outer walls resembling onion skin.

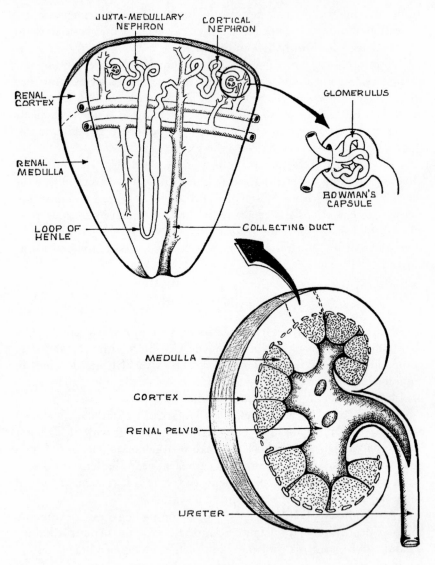

Kidney Structure

The presence of immune system complexes consisting of antigen, antibody and complement is also related to kidney disease and a poorer outcome. Patients with lupus are likely to have elevated concentrations of lupus anticoagulant, an antiphospholipid antibody that predisposes them to thrombosis (including strokes, pulmonary embolus, and deep vein thrombosis) and miscarriage. Thirty percent of patients with lupus

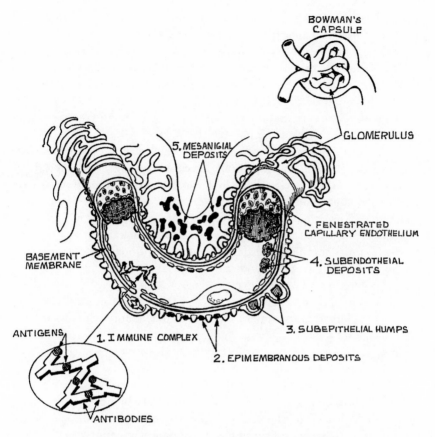

BOWMAN'S
CAPSULE

GLOMERULUS

5. MESANIGIAL
DEPOSITS

FENESTRATED
CAPILLARY ENDOTHELIUM

BASEMENT
MEMBRANE

4. SUBENDOTHEIAL
DEPOSITS

ANTIGENS

1. IMMUNE COMPLEX

3. SUBEPITHELIAL HUMPS

2. EPIMEMBRANOUS DEPOSITS

ANTIBODIES

Immune Complexes in Autoimmune Kidney Disease

anticoagulant will exhibit abnormalities in routine blood coagulation tests.

Rheumatologists avoid prescribing oral contraceptives or estrogen replacement therapy for women with lupus because of the widely held view that estrogen can aggravate the disease. The National Institutes of Health is currently conducting clinical trials on the safety of estrogens in SLE.

Lupus Nephritis

The kidney involvement that affects approximately 50 percent of patients with SLE is called lupus nephritis. Kidneys normally function to remove toxic metabolites and drugs and to control the tonicity, volume and chemical composition of urine. The basic unit of the kidney is the renal tubule or nephron. Each kidney has about one million nephrons, and each nephron contains a filtering system known as a glomerulus, and a tubule, through which the filtered urine passes.

The glomerulus is a lobulated network of convoluted capillary vessels held together by scanty connective tissue. This capillary network is derived from a small arterial twig, the afferent vessel, which enters the capsule, generally at a point opposite to that at which the latter is connected with the tubule, and the resulting vein, the efferent vessel, emerges from the capsule at the same point.

The glomerular or Bowman's capsule, which surrounds the glomerulus, consists of a basement membrane, lined on its inner surface by a layer of flattened epithelial cells. The whole surface of the glomerulus is covered with a continuous layer of the same cells, on a delicate supporting membrane. Normally, blood flows into glomerulus, and while it's in the capillaries, waste materials are forced out and minerals are reabsorbed. When immune complexes or deposits of IgA antibodies clog the filtration system, protein and blood can escape along with the waste. The excess protein loss causes edema.

Lupus nephritis primarily affects the glomeruli causing cellular proliferations, glomerular basement membrane thickening, white blood cell infiltration and sclerosis. These changes may involve all of the glomeruli (diffuse), a minority of glomeruli (focal), a part of each glomerulus (segmental), or predominately the mesangium (mesangial).

The fulminant fatal renal glomerular disease of SLE (diffuse proliferative nephritis) is characterized by fine punctate hemorrhages dotting the cortical surface of the kidney. These hemorrhages are caused by inflammatory damage and rupture of the glomerular capillaries.

Neuropsychiatric SLE (NPSLE)

Neurologic or psychiatric abnormalities may occur in up to two-thirds of patients with SLE.[3] Although there are no widely accepted diagnostic criteria established for NPSLE, the clinical manifestations are reported to range from cognitive dysfunction to life-threatening crises. NPSLE is defined as a significant and unequivocal change in baseline neurologic and psychiatric function identified by history and physical examination.

In most patients NPSLE develops within the first two years of the onset of SLE, although it can occur at any time. The disease mechanism consists of (1) primary events related to the effects of autoantibodies on the nervous system and, more commonly, (2) secondary events that result indirectly from other organ system lesions, such as kidney disease with hypertension, uremia, complications of therapy or superficial infections.

Organic brain syndromes are the most common manifestation of NPSLE and may affect 50 percent of SLE patients during the course of their disease.[4] Symptoms of organic brain syndrome include impairment of memory, intellect and judgment, as well as delirium. Other symptoms of NPSLE include seizures, headache, cranial and peripheral neuropathies, strokes, and movement disorders.

Autoantibodies in NPSLE

Antineuronal antibody levels in the cerebrospinal fluid (CSF) are generally present in active central nervous system disease. Antineuronal antibody titers are much higher in the CSF of patients with active nervous system involvement when compared to SLE patients free of neuropsychiatric symptoms. Levels of interferon-alpha and interleukin-2 are also higher in the CSF of patients with NPSLE, and over-expression of pro-inflammatory cytokines is commonly seen.

Antibodies directed against ribosomal P protein are also seen in most SLE patients with organic psychosis compared to 10 percent to 20 percent of SLE patients without neuropsychiatric disorders. And while about 20 percent of SLE patients have antiphospholipid antibodies, up to 55 percent of patients with NPSLE have antiphospholipid antibodies.[5]

A LINK TO SCHIZOPHRENIA?

Increased prevalence of antinuclear antibodies and also antibodies targeted against neurotransmitters (chemicals which send messages between the immune and endocrine system) and platelets (blood components necessary for clotting) have been found in schizophrenia. Other immunologic abnormalities seen in schizophrenia include altered cytokine levels and increased levels of soluble cytokine receptors.

RHEUMATOID ARTHRITIS

Rheumatoid arthritis (RA) is a widespread chronic system inflammatory disease characterized by polyarthritis that may be progressive and permanently deforming. RA affects about 1 percent of the population. Its primary target is women, who are affected three times as often as men.

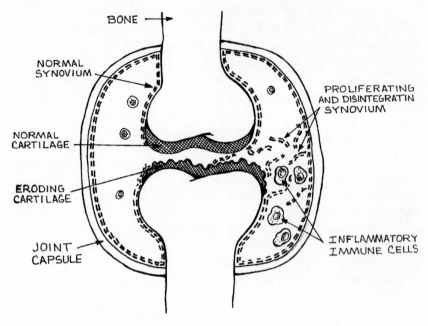

Autoimmune Effects on Synovium in Rheumatoid Arthritis

In RA, joint pain and inflammation occur symmetrically, affecting both sides of the body equally. RA targets joints in the fingers, wrists, elbows, shoulders, neck, jaws, knees, ankles, hips and feet. RA is characterized by chronic proliferative and inflammatory changes in the synovial membrane (interior of joint capsule lined by cells called synoviocytes) accompanied by inflammatory effusion in the joint space, which may lead to destruction of articular cartilage. Ultimately, the joint space becomes obliterated and the bone ends united (ankylosis).

In advanced arthritis, virtually all of the articular cartilage is replaced by rheumatoid inflammatory membrane. One nonviable remnant of eroded cartilage remains attached to the subchondral bone, and fragments of cartilage become embedded in the inflammatory membrane.

Other Symptoms Associated with RA

Extra-articular manifestations (symptoms associated with other organs besides the joints) include rheumatoid nodules (granulomatosus tissue growths, occurring subcutaneously or directly under the skin, particularly in the tendon, lungs and heart), pericarditis, and arteritis.

RA is known to involve the heart in 20 percent to 40 percent of cases of severe prolonged disease. The most common finding is pericarditis, an inflammation of the sac surrounding the heart that may progress to fibrous thickening of the pericardium and its adhesions. In the early stages of this process, inflammatory nodules may occur on the pericardial surfaces or the heart valves.

Genetic and Immunologic Components

The HLA antigen DR4 described in chapter 4 is seen in 65 percent to 60 percent of patients with RA. Its presence is usually related to more severe symptoms. In RA, autoantibodies to the crystallizable fraction of IgG cause inflammation. Typically, the synovial or joint fluid contains high concentrations of white blood cells. In active rheumatoid arthritis, rheumatoid factor (RF) as well as the erythrocyte sedimentation rate (ESR) are elevated.

While inflammation often results from aggregates consisting of white blood cells and RF, RF complexes with IgG may be formed locally, in synovial fluid, or in the circulation. These complexes may activate complement, neutrophil, and macrophage-mediated mechanisms of joint and extrarticular injury and inflammation.

Cell-mediated mechanisms and pro-inflammatory cytokines, particularly tissue necrosis factor-alpha, a significant promoter of joint inflammation, are also associated with symptoms in RA. Lymphocytes, primarily T helper lymphocytes, many of which are activated, are the most abundant cells in the rheumatoid synovial membrane. Many activated blood and tissue cells capable of expressing HLA-DR antigen are also present.

Levels of IL-15 and IL-17 have also been recently found to be elevated in the synovium (fluid-filled cavity surrounding the joint) of patients with RA. Both of these cytokines are known to trigger cascades of pro-inflammatory cytokines that likely contribute to symptoms in RA.

Environmental Triggers

One recent study described the role of the bacteria *Salmonella* in triggering RA development. Researchers found that the immune system cells that fight bacteria can also attack normal cells that are carrying a specific protein that resembles bacterial protein.[6]

In patients infected with *Salmonella* food poisoning, approximately 10 percent go on to develop a reactive type of arthritis. But a smaller number of those patients get a severe long-lasting type of arthritis. Furthermore, previously infected individuals who have mild initial responses and are later re-infected are likely to develop RA through a process of molecular mimicry.

POLYARTERITIS NODOSA

In polyarteritis disorders, the arteries of any of the major organs may be affected with vasculitis (inflammation of blood vessels). Pathologically, polyarteritis is characterized by cellular destruction and a white blood cell infiltration of all three layers that make up the blood vessel wall.

Polyarteritis nodosa (PAN) is a classical model of systemic, noninfectious, necrotizing (cell or tissue destroying) vasculitis that involves small and medium sized arteries of the kidney. The entire wall of the small artery is the site of acute necrosis and neutrophilic white blood cell infiltration in both the vessel wall and surrounding tissue. Many of the epithelial cells that line blood vessels are detached and displaced, contributing to the possibility of clots (thrombosis) and arterial blockages.

Environmental Triggers

Up to 20 percent to 30 percent of patients with polyarteritis have hepatitis B virus antigens. Hepatitis B surface antigens and antigen complexes are present in the circulation and deposited in the vascular lesions of patients with these disorders, suggesting that this virus is a trigger for polyarteritis.

DERMATOMYOSITIS

Dermatomyositis is an inflammatory disease affecting the skin and muscles. Typical symptoms include a purplish swelling around the eyes commonly referred to as heliotrope rash, red papules over the knuckles known as Gottron's papules, redness or atrophy in areas of the skin exposed to the sun, scaling of the scalp, palms and soles, hair loss, and redness and blood vessel changes around the nails.

Muscle involvement in dermatomyositis typically causes weakness or fatigue and primarily affects the muscles closest to the trunk, such as those of the shoulders and hip. Patients may also develop heart conduction disorders, lung inflammation, weakening of the diaphragm and difficulty swallowing.

Biopsies are generally used to confirm the diagnosis of dermatomyositis. Granular antibody complex deposits are typically found between the epidermal and dermal layers of skin lesions. Most patients also have positive ANA titers and antibodies to the enzyme Jo-1. Since cancer is present in up to 25 percent of patients with dermatomyositis, tests for tumor markers and CAT scans are also included in the diagnostic workup.

ATHEROSCLEROSIS

There is significant evidence that an autoimmune response is involved in atherosclerosis. Increased levels of autoantibodies to heat shock protein 65/60, gangliosides, and oxidized low-density lipoproteins have been demonstrated in atherosclerotic lesions. Furthermore, these lesions were found to have elevated levels of MHC class II expression and increased levels of certain cytokines.

Environmental Triggers

Heat shock protein 65/60 is considered by some researchers to be the most likely autoantigen trigger for the autoimmune response in atherosclerosis. In animal studies, immunization with this antigen has been found to precipitate the development of atherosclerotic lesions in the aorta of rabbits.[7]

PEMPHIGOID DISORDERS

Pemphigus (from the Greek pemphix, meaning bubble or blister) encompasses a group of autoimmune skin diseases characterized by severe bullae or blistering of the epidermis and mucous membranes. The most

common pemphigus disorders are (1) pemphigus vulgaris, a disorder that
destroys epidermal skin up to the suprabasilar level and (2) pemphigus
foliaceus, which destroys epidermal skin at the subcorneal levels. Both disorders were usually fatal before the introduction of glucocorticoid therapy. Other pemphigoid disorders include paraneoplastic pemphigus,
which is associated with lymphoma, and drug-induced pemphigus, which
usually develops after the administration of the drug penicillamine.

Pemphigus primarily affects adults in mid-life and primarily occurs
in individuals of eastern European Jewish ancestry and in patients from
northern India and Asia.

Immunology

Patients with pemphigus vulgaris have autoantibodies that bind to the
surface of keratinocytes, the cells that form the epidermis. In pemphigus
foliaceus autoantibodies target keratinocytes in the subcorneal region. Both
of these autoantibodies are specifically directed at the desmoglein glyco-
porteins that form cell-adhesion molecules. The structural integrity of the
epidermis normally depends on the sharing of desmoglein protein by
neighboring skin cells. Although pemphigoid mothers can pass autoantibodies to their offspring, newborns have a different composition of
desmoglein types, and, consequently, remain unaffected.

Environmental Triggers

Studies in rural areas of South America and Tunisia suggest that
pemphigoid disorders can be triggered in susceptible individuals by a form
of antigenic mimicry that occurs between desmoglein and an unidentified
infectious agent. These endemic pemphigoid disorders are clinically identical to the usual pemphigoid disorders.

AUTOIMMUNE THYROID DISEASES

Autoimmune thyroid disease (AITD) includes a number of different
disorders affecting thyroid function, resulting in low thyroid hormone
levels (hypothyroidism) or excess thyroid hormone production (hyperthyroidism). Some patients with AITD may be euthyroid (normal blood

hormone levels) but have the associated eye disorder known as Graves' ophthalmopathy.

Normally, thyroid hormone levels are regulated by the pituitary hormone, thyrotropin stimulating hormone (TSH). Thyroid autoantibodies that target the TSH receptor in AITDs can cause excess stimulation of thyroid hormone or they can block TSH at the receptor, causing hypothyroidism. AITD patients have a combination of thyroid antibodies, with the predominant antibody causing the primary symptoms.

Cytotoxic lymphocytes and other thyroid antibodies, including thyroglobulin, thyroid peroxidase and thyroid growth immunoglobulins cause thyroid cell damage, growth, and inflammation, and also contribute to the disease process in AITDs.

Symptoms

Cardiac symptoms are among the earliest features of both hyperthyroidism and hypothyroidism. In hyperthyroidism, tachycardia, palpitations and enlarged heart are common, and arrhythmias occasionally appear. In hypothyroidism, cardiac output is decreased, with reduced stroke volume and heart rate and there is decreased blood flow to peripheral tissues. Reduced circulation in the skin accounts for the characteristic cold sensitivity. In advanced myxedema, the heart is flabby, enlarged and dilated.

Environmental Triggers

Iodine, infectious agents, especially viruses, pesticides, estrogens and stress are known environmental triggers of autoimmune thyroid disease. Beef contaminated with thyroid hormone, stress, for instance stress associated with the loss of a parent or time spent in concentration camps, and diet supplements containing iodine and thyroid hormone precursors such as TRIAC and TETRAC are all associated with mini-epidemics of Graves' disease.

INSULIN DEPENDENT DIABETES MELLITUS

In the United States, the rates of IDDM are increasing. Between 12,000 and 14,000 children and adolescents are diagnosed with insulin dependent diabetes mellitus (IDDM) each year. IDDM is half as common in African-American children as in white children. In Asian Americans and Native Americans, IDDM is rare. However, while IDDM affects approximately one in every 300 to 500 Americans, IDDM affects one in 100 Scandinavians, especially Swedes and Finns.[8]

IDDM is responsible for both macrovascular and microvascular disease symptoms. Macrovascular diseases include (1) carotid artery disease, including stroke, (2) coronary artery disease, including heart attacks, and (3) peripheral vascular disease, including claudication or decreased blood flow to blood vessels in the legs, and blockages of the extremities resulting in gangrene (the death of tissue owing to ischemia or lack of oxygen). In the United States, gangrene associated with IDDM is the leading cause of lower extremity amputation.

Microvascular disease damages the blood vessels of the eyes (retinopathy) and kidneys (nephropathy which may progress to renal failure). The extent of capillary damage is directly proportion to the severity and duration of hyperglycemia (elevated blood sugar). Diabetic retinopathy is the leading cause of blindness in the United States, and diabetic nephropathy is the leading cause of renal failure.

Immunology and Genetics

IDDM results from chronic autoimmune destruction of the insulin-producing beta cells in the pancreas. The autoimmune mechanism involves a cell-mediated attack on the pancreatic islets and autoantibody formation. Family history is a strong predictive factor with the HLA alleles B8, B15, and B18 showing susceptibility for IDDM when they're in linkage disequilibrium with HLA DR3 and DR4.

More than 20 separate autoantibody markers for IDDM have been found, including ICA, insulin receptor antibodies, islet cells surface antibodies (ISCA) and glutamic acid decarboxylase antibodies. ICA titers are commonly expressed in JDF (Juvenile Diabetes Foundation) units. Low titers may spontaneously revert to negative. However, high titers (greater than 20 units) only rarely revert to negative.

With the knowledge that autoantibodies to beta cells are responsible for impaired insulin production in IDDM, several studies in the 1980s focused on the use of immunosuppresants to curb autoantibody production. Transient remission was seen in 50 percent of patients. However, in most instances the white blood cell suppression caused by these drugs prohibited their routine use. Furthermore, it was found that treatment in

IDDM could only be effective if it halted autoantibody production prior to extensive beta cell destruction and necrosis.

Environmental Triggers

In IDDM genetically susceptible individuals are exposed to environmental triggers that initiate the formation of autoantibodies that target insulin-secreting pancreatic islet and beta cells.

Discussions of environmental triggers have focused upon diet, environmental exposures, particularly to bovine albumin in cow's milk, and viral infections. Viral infections are known to cause insulin resistance, which increases the body's demands for insulin. While some studies have shown the presence of Coxsackie B virus in the pancreatic cells of children with IDDM, most cases of IDDM show no evidence of this virus. Other viruses implicated in IDDM include Coxsackie A, cytomegalovirus, echo virus, Epstein-Barr virus, rubella, mumps, and retroviruses.[9]

In September 2000, Dr. J. Barthelow Classen, Director of Classen Immunotherapies, presented data at the International Public Conference on Vaccination, which implicated vaccines as the primary cause of IDDM in children. Classen's data include the pertussis, mumps, rubella, hepatitis B, and haemophilus vaccines.[10]

Treatment

Treatment for IDDM today focuses on prevention, which involves recognizing prediabetes. The most promising preventive measures involve a mechanism known as tolerization. In oral tolerance therapy, the autoantigen targeted by insulin antibodies is administered orally or injected. The goal here is to develop a suppressive or tolerant immune response in individuals determined to be at risk by virtue of genetic prescreening and islet autoantibody testing.[11] Initially used as an alternative medicine therapy, oral tolerance therapy is the focus of current clinical trials.

AUTOIMMUNE LIVER DISORDERS

The largest of the body's organs, the liver is responsible for more than six hundred metabolic functions, including metabolizing glucose, proteins and hormones, synthesizing bile, and storing nutrients. The liver receives blood directly from both the gastrointestinal tract and the systemic circulation.

In its function of processing blood, the liver removes toxins and ammonia and breaks them down into less harmful substances. The liver also processes and stores nutrients, including fat-soluble vitamins, folate, vitamin B12 and minerals such as copper and iron. When the liver is diseased, dying liver cells release enzymes, which, along with toxins and ammonia, accumulate in the blood. Consequently, blood levels of liver enzymes are elevated in liver disease.

Autoimmune liver diseases may be hepatic or cholestatic in nature. Hepatic diseases include chronic autoimmune hepatitis (CAH), a disorder in which the liver's functional cells, the hepatocytes, are targeted. Cholestatic diseases include diseases such as primary biliary cirrhosis (PBC) or autoimmune cholangitis, diseases responsible for the blockage of bile flow and which eventually result in destruction of bile ducts. Overlap syndromes may also be present, in which the patient has both hepatic and cholestatic disorders.

Liver Function

Produced by hepatocytes, bile is a greenish fluid that consists of cholesterol, phospholipids, bilirubin (the breakdown product of hemoglobin which occurs when red blood cells die), and bile salts. Bile salts act as detergents since they aid in the digestion and absorption of dietary fats. After leaving the liver via bile ducts, bile is temporarily stored in the gallbladder. From there bile is emptied into the small intestine.

Symptoms

Symptoms of liver disease include decreased appetite, nausea, vomiting, jaundice, pruritus (itching), skin xanthomas, edema, ascites (abdominal edema), and metabolic bone changes including osteoporosis. The pruritus associated with liver disease is usually treated with cholestyramine.

Autoimmune liver disease is suspected whenever symptoms of liver disease are present and blood or imaging tests show certain abnormalities. Blood liver function tests include measurements of liver enzymes and the compounds normally synthesized by the liver, including proteins and the clotting factor prothrombin. Serum bilirubin (the deep yellow compound responsible for jaundice) levels are rarely elevated at the onset of the disease, but they eventually rise as the disease progresses.

Tests for viral antibodies to hepatitis A, B, C, and D are commonly measured to rule out viral hepatitis. In autoimmune hepatitis, viral antibody titers are typically negative. However, autoimmune liver disease may develop in patients with previously diagnosed cases of hepatitis C.

Globulin levels are increased and albumin is decreased in both hepatic and cholestatic autoimmune liver disorders. Hyaluronan is increased in cirrhotic liver disorders, while haptoglobin is decreased in most types of liver disease.

Immunology

Autoantibodies associated with autoimmune liver disease include: antinuclear (ANA) antibodies, antimitochondrial (AMA) antibodies, anti-smooth muscle (ASMA) antibodies, anti-double stranded (ds)DNA, anti-neutrophil cytoplasmic abs (ANCA), anti-soluble liver antigens (SLA), anti-liver/kidney microsomes (ALKM-1), and anti-liver cytosol antigen (ALC-2).

Positive titers for ANA and ASMA are seen in type 1 autoimmune hepatitis and primary biliary cirrhosis. A positive SLA and dsDNA are seen in type 1 hepatitis A. Positive AMA (>20) is seen in primary biliary cirrhosis. A positive ANCA is seen in primary sclerosing cholangitis and type 1 autoimmune hepatitis. A positive ALC-1 and sometimes ALKM-1 are seen in type 2 autoimmune hepatitis. Note: ALKM-2 and ALKM-3 are also seen in non-autoimmune forms of hepatitis. HLA antigens A1/B8/DR3 are associated with autoimmune hepatitis.

Chronic autoimmune hepatitis

Autoimmune hepatitis occurs as two distinct subtypes, type 1 and type 2. Both disorders are characterized by an inflammatory process and hepatocyte destruction, and both types are seen more often in women. Both disorders also respond well to immunosupressant medications. Autoimmune hepatitis may occur in association with other autoimmune diseases, including Crohn's disease, thyroiditis, and Sjögren's syndrome. Autoimmune hepatitis may accompany the autoimmune liver disorders

PBC and PSC (described below), and this overlapping syndrome may be more common than previously thought.

Primary Biliary Cirrhosis

Primary Biliary Cirrhosis (PBC) is the most frequently seen autoimmune cholestatic disorder. PBC primarily occurs in middle-aged women, and its incidence has increased in recent years, with PBC now reported to occur in 94 out of 100,100 women older than 40. PBC is characterized by damage or destruction of interlobular and proximal bile ducts. More than 98 percent of patients with PBC have positive antimitochondrial antibody (AMA) titers. PBC may occur as a primary disorder or it may accompany almost any of the other autoimmune disorders. Approximately 4 percent of patients with PBC also have scleroderma.

Gallstones, usually of pigment type, occur in nearly 40 percent of cases. Liver biopsy indicates bile duct damage. Other symptoms include finger clubbing, and occasionally osteoarthropathy is present. About 20 percent of patients with PBC are reported to have autoimmune thyroiditis, including Graves' disease. And 25 percent of patients with GD have low titers of anti-mitochondrial antibodies for no apparent reason.

Autoimmune cholangitis

Symptoms of autoimmune cholangitis are similar to those of PBC. However, the immunological picture is different. Patients with cholangitis do not have AMA.

A subtype of cholangitis known as primary sclerosing cholangitis (PSC) affects both the intra- and extrahepatic biliary trees, resulting in a chronic, fibrosing, inflammatory process which results in obliteration of the biliary tree and ultimate biliary cirrhosis. PSC is associated with inflammatory bowel disease, and it occurs more frequently in men than women.

Symptoms include weight loss, fatigue, right upper quadrant abdominal pain, pruritis (itching), and intermittent jaundice. Circulating immune complexes contribute to the bile duct destruction seen in this disease. Further evidence of the autoimmune nature of this disease is its association with the HLA antigens B8 and DR3.

AUTOIMMUNE
INFLAMMATORY BOWEL DISEASE

Inflammatory bowel disease (IBD) refers to idiopathic inflammatory conditions of the bowel, mainly ulcerative colitis, Crohn's disease, and celiac disease. Typically, patients with IBD have symptoms of diarrhea, abdominal pain and fecal blood loss.

Ulcerative Colitis

Ulcerative colitis primarily involves the mucosal lining of the colon. Typically, the disease involves the rectum and the entire colon. Ulcerative colitis is associated with an increased risk for the development of colon cancer.

Crohn's Disease

Crohn's disease may involve any part of the intestines including the colon. Often, the entire bowel wall is involved. Inflammatory cytokines are thought to play a role in perpetuating the inflammation seen in this disorder. In one study, eight of ten patients who had no response to conventional therapy went into remission after a single dose of a monoclonal antibody targeting the cytokine TNF-alpha.[12]

Immunology

The key feature in IBD is inflammation with lesions showing immune involvement. The lesions typically seen in ulcerative colitis resemble those caused by antigen-antibody complexes. However, there are no studies that can conclusively prove an association with immune complexes.

Anticolon antibodies are typically seen in patients with IBD, but these autoantibodies are not diagnostic since they are also seen in patients with cirrhosis and urinary tract infections. Perinuclear antineutrophil cytoplasmic antibodies (P-ANCA) are also associated with IBD. Fifty percent to 90 percent of patients with ulcerative colitis have atypical P-ANCA.

Environmental Triggers

Although several microorganisms have been proposed as etiologic agents in IBD, there are no data that definitively point to one particular agent.

NEUROLOGICAL AND
NEUROMUSCULAR DISORDERS

Autoimmune Encephalomyelitis

Autoimmune encephalomyelitis is a rare nervous system disorder characterized by inflammation of the brain and spinal cord. According to researchers at the Natural Toxins Research Center at Texas A&M University in Kingsville, this disorder is becoming more common because of the practice of vaccination.

Immunology

One example is the reaction to certain types of rabies vaccine, particularly those using the Pasteur treatment. Here, the rabies virus was injected into a rabbit, where the organism proliferated in the brain and spinal cord. This virus was extracted and inactivated, and then administered to the patient as a vaccine. In some instances, an immune reaction against myelin in neural tissues resulted, causing autoimmune encephalomyelitis in the vaccinated individual.[13]

Environmental Triggers

Although this type of rabies vaccine is rarely used today, a similar response can be seen with other vaccines. Depending on the source of live vaccine, the inactivated virus can be contaminated with host brain antigens, causing encephalomyelitis and a number of other vaccine associated adverse effects (VAAEs).[14]

Multiple Sclerosis (MS)

Multiple sclerosis (MS) is one of the leading causes of chronic neurological disability in young adults. MS is more frequently seen in

Caucasians than in African Americans and Asians. Caucasians of northern European ancestry have the greatest chances of developing MS.

In MS, T lymphocytes along with autoantibodies to myelin basic protein randomly attack and destroy the myelin protective sheath that insulates and protects nerves in the brain and spinal cord. Denuded, these nerves lose the ability to transmit messages normally. Depending on which areas of the nervous system are involved, symptoms may be mild or severe, involving multiple organ systems.

Symptoms

Typical symptoms include impairment of vision, balance, coordination and mobility as well as decreased sexual activity, and loss of bowel and bladder control. Despite these limitations, with treatment approximately 75 percent of MS patients remain ambulatory (able to walk without assisting devices) for life, and mental faculties generally remain intact.

While most cases of MS appear to have an autoimmune origin, there appears to be an identical form of MS in which there is no immune system involvement. Most experts believe that a virus is ultimately responsible for both forms of MS. The causative agent, which has not yet been identified, apparently takes root in the first 15 years of life.[15]

Although many of the symptoms of MS are similar to those of other disorders, a careful neurological exam generally shows a delayed to response to visual stimuli. Analysis of the spinal fluid may reveal increased amounts of protein caused by the degradation of myelin. An MRI is also helpful in detecting early neurological changes.

Environmental Triggers

Doctors frequently warn patients with MS to avoid high temperatures. Heat has been found to further delay the conduction of electrical impulses in diseased nerves, aggravating symptoms. Cold temperatures, on the other hand, increase the velocity of impulses. Patients with MS generally benefit from exercising in cold water. Physical therapy and exercise can maintain muscle strength and improve coordination.

Gamma-interferon used in therapy is known to induce the development of MS. A link between Epstein-Barr virus, which causes infectious mononucleosis, is also being explored. Patients with both disorders have abnormally low levels of essential fatty acids and Vitamin D.

Guillain-Barré Syndrome

Guillain-Barré syndrome (GBS), an AD that targets the myelin sheath covering the nerves, affects about 2,000 to 3,000 Americans annually. Its onset is sudden and symptoms typically progress quickly. Although the exact cause has not been determined, GBS often occurs shortly after viral infections and vaccinations, specifically vaccinations against measles, mumps, and the influenza virus.[16] GBS may also flare up during pregnancy, following surgery or, rarely, during another serious illness.

The sensory and motor systems of afflicted patients may be equally affected. However, the primary disorder is a demyelinating polyneuorpathy characterized by a gradual diminishment of muscular strength and motor paralysis. Limbs are typically flaccid and patients do not exhibit spasms or seizures. The onset of paralysis is often preceded by a general feeling of weakness. Patients frequently mention experiencing cramps or a pins and needles sensation in their hands and feet before paralysis sets in.

The limbs, particularly the lower limbs, are affected first. Symptoms can range from mild to severe to fatal, depending on the extent of damage to the insulating myelin sheath covering the nerves. In some instances, the entire muscular system, including the muscles of the respiratory system, may be affected.

Immunology

An evaluation for ganglioside autoantibodies is typically used to aid in the diagnosis of GBS. Typically, antibodies that target myelin are seen in GBS.

Environmental Triggers and Treatment

Molecular mimicry between various viral, bacterial and parasitic antigens is known to precipitate the development of ganglioside autoantibodies. Infection with Cytomegalovirus (CMV) and also Campylobacter jejuni are often implicated. Antecedent CMV and Campylobacter infections are also associated with a poorer prognosis.[17] Highest frequencies of myelin-specific autoantibodies in GBS are seen against the gangliosides sulfatide and cardiolipin.

Drugs such as prednisone, that are used to treat other autoimmune disorders are ineffective in Guillain-Barré and may even be harmful. About 5 percent of patients die, and 5 to 15 percent have lasting disabilities. But after treatment, which typically lasts for three months to a year, 50 percent to 90 percent of patients recover fully or exhibit only mild abnormalities. GBS usually spontaneously resolves although patients with recurrences often develop the autoimmune disorder chronic inflammatory demyelinating polyneuropathy (CIDP). In the related cranial disorder known as Miller-Fisher syndrome, neuropathy is specific for the cranial region.

Myasthenia Gravis (MG)

The name myasthenia gravis means "grave muscle weakness" in reference to the profound skeletal muscle weakness and fatigue characteristic of this disorder. If the respiratory muscles are affected, MG can be fatal. Although the cause of MG is unknown, the basic abnormality is a reduction in the number of acetylcholine receptors found on muscle membranes at the neuromuscular junction. This reduction is caused by autoantoantibodies that target and destroy the acetylcholine receptor.

Normally, skeletal muscle cells are innervated by motor neurons that release the neurotransmitter acetylcholine into the neuromuscular junction where it diffuses over to the muscle membrane. When acetylcholine receptors on muscle cells are loaded with this neurotransmitter, they can counteract the cholinesterase enzyme and initiate a signal that induces skeletal muscle contraction. In MG, this normal functioning is impaired, leading to aberrant muscle contraction.

Immunology

Furthermore, the acetylcholinesterase receptor antibodies can activate complement, form immune complexes, promote cellular toxicity responses, and directly destroy acetylcholine receptors. If enough receptors are destroyed, muscle contraction cannot be triggered unless cholinesterase activity is also inhibited, allowing the remaining receptor sites to be continually stimulated by acetylcholine.

AUTOIMMUNE POLYGLANDULAR (POLYENDOCRINE) SYNDROMES

Autoimmune diseases occasionally occur as cluster syndromes. In these cluster syndromes, two or more autoimmune endocrine diseases coexist within the same patient.

In the autoimmune polyglandular (polyendocrine) syndromes, patients are affected by a certain specific cluster of endocrine disorders that have a tendency to occur together. All of the organs or glands involved in the polyglandular syndromes are characterized by a mononuclear (lymphocytes and macrophages) cell infiltration that targets specific tissues, while sparing their surrounding components.

For instance, in Addison's disease (adrenal gland insufficiency), a member of the type 1 polyglandular group, the adrenal cortex (of the adrenal gland) shows marked cellular infiltration and cell destruction while the adrenal medulla remains unaffected. Chronic autoimmune or Hashimoto's thyroiditis is frequently seen in patients with type 2 and type 3 polyglandular syndrome. Eventually, all of the organs affected by the polyglandular syndromes undergo fibrosis and atrophy as all of their functional endocrine cells are destroyed.

Type 1 autoimmune polyglandular syndrome

Type 1 autoimmune polyglandular syndrome includes hypoparathyroidism, adrenal insufficiency and candidiasis (yeast infection). Type 1 polyglandular syndrome generally emerges in children before age 10 and is manifested by a skin disorder as well as the yeast infection known as candidiasis. Typically, hypoparathyroidism emerges next, followed by Addison's disease, an adrenal deficiency disorder, a few years later.

Up to 20 percent of patients with Addison's disease have premature gonadal failure, and a significant number of those have steroidal cell antibodies directed against cytochrome P enzymes, causing lymphocytic infiltration of the ovaries. Autoimmune oophoritis may cause primary amenorrhea (absence of menstrual periods) or the disorder may emerge long after menarche (after the first menstrual period), resulting in secondary amenorrhea preceded by progressive oligomenorrhea (scant menstrual periods).[18]

Type 2 autoimmune polyglandular syndrome

Type 2 autoimmune polyglandular syndrome (also known as Schmidt's syndrome) is characterized by adrenal insufficiency occurring concomitantly with either autoimmune thyroid disease or type 1 diabetes. Other conditions seen as part of the type 2 polyglandular syndrome include premature ovarian failure, myasthenia gravis, celiac disease, alopecia, hypophysitis, vitiligo, serositis, and pernicious anemia.

Type 3 autoimmune polyglandular syndrome

Type 3 autoimmune polyglandular syndrome involves autoimmune thyroid disease, usually Hashimoto's thyroiditis, and at least two other ADs, excluding Addison's disease (adrenal insufficiency). Besides autoimmune thyroid disease, patients with type 3 polyglandular syndrome commonly have coexisting conditions of insulin dependent diabetes mellitus, pernicious anemia, or other organ specific ADs such as myasthenia gravis.

AUTOIMMUNE REPRODUCTIVE DISORDERS

Autoimmune Oophritis

The autoimmune ovarian disorder oophritis may occur in conjunction with other autoimmune endocrine disorders, especially Addison's disease, or it may emerge as a primary disorder. In oophritis, a number of structural ovarian abnormalities occur. Lymphocytes and plasma cells infiltrate growing ovarian follicles, corpora lutea, and other endocrine cells. Antibodies to ovarian cells known as oocytes are often seen. The target appears to be the maturing ovarian follicles rather than the primordial follicles. The active inflammatory phase of this disorder is transient. After an extended period of amenorrhea, the ovaries may appear small and atrophied with few or no follicles.

Chronic Orchitis

Orchitis, an autoimmune disorder affecting males and causing infertility, is characterized by antibodies to sperm or by lymphocytic infiltration of spermatazoa.

Environmental Triggers

Rupture or trauma, including vasectomy, is reported to account for the presence of sperm antibodies.

Peyronie's Disease

Peyronie's disease is a localized connective tissue disorder of the tunica albuginea, the whitish membrane within the penis that surrounds the spongy chambers, helping to trap blood, which is needed to sustain erection. Symptoms include painful erections and curvature of the penis.

Genetics and Environmental Triggers

Peyronie's disease is associated with the HLA antigen DRw52, and studies indicate dysregulation of wound healing related to repetitive microtrauma incurred during intercourse is a probable cause.[19]

AUTOIMMUNE HEMOLYTIC ANEMIA (AIHA)

Autoimmune hemolytic anemia includes several disorders that are characterized by autoantibodies that can to bind to the blood group antigens of erythrocytes (red blood cells). Autoimmune anemias that are not drug induced fall into two major categories, warm and cold, depending on the temperature at which they optimally react.

The binding of warm antibody to erythrocytes causes the rapid clearance of sensitized erythrocytes in the spleen, which causes anemia. Cold reactive autoantibodies can bind, fix complement and cause hemolysis (red cell lysis or destruction) in areas of the peripheral circulation where peripheral circulation temperatures fall below 37° C. Agglutination can also occur, causing tissue destruction and blockages in the extremities. Complement-mediated hemolysis can also occur, provoking intravascular lesions.

Environmental Triggers

Drug-induced AIHA occurs when certain drugs act as haptens and bind with erythrocyte antigens, inducing autoantibody formation. These autoantibodies bind to erythrocytes, causing hemagglutination or hemolysis, which leads to anemia.

CHAGAS' DISEASE AND PARASITIC INFECTIONS

Chagas' disease, which is also known as American trypanosomiasis, is directly caused by *Trypanosoma cruzi*, a protozoan parasite. Chagas' disease is the most frequent cause of heart failure in Brazil and neighboring Latin American countries. *T. cruzi* parasites are transmitted from person to person via "kissing bugs," which hide in the cracks of houses, feed on the sleeping inhabitants, and pass infectious parasites in the feces. These parasites enter the host through damaged skin or through mucous membranes. At the site of entry, there may be a transient reddened nodule called a chagoma.

In acute Chagas' disease, cardiac damage results from the direct invasion of myocardial cells by the infectious agent and from the resultant inflammatory process. Chronic Chagas' disease affects 20 percent of infected patients approximately 5 to 15 years after the initial infection. An autoimmune response induced by *T. cruzi* parasites damages the heart and digestive tract.

Patients with Chagas' disease have antibodies and T cells that react with parasite proteins and cross-react with host myocardial and nerve cells, lymphocytes and extracellular proteins. Damage to myocardial cells and to conductance pathways results in heart muscle damage (cardiomyopathy) and disturbances in heart rhythm (cardiac arrhythmias). Digestive tract changes include dilation of both the colon and esophagus.[20]

VASCULITIS AND ARTERITIS

Inflammation of the blood vessels, often with necrosis or tissue destruction, is called vasculitis or arteritis. The terms are generally used interchangeably because veins and capillaries may also be involved. Immune-mediated inflammation is one of the most common causes of these disorders. Immune complexes are responsible for the vascular lesions seen in SLE associated vasculitis. In patients with mixed cryoglobulinemia, immunoglobulins and complement have been found in involved vessels.

Antineutrophil cytoplasmic autoantibodies (ANCA) are responsible for the vasculitis seen in Wegener's granulomatosis and microscopic polyangiitis. The titers of these antibodies usually correlate with disease severity. It's thought that these antibodies activate neutrophils, stimulating the release of toxic oxygen free radicals and also enzymes capable of cell lysis. This neutrophil activation is also potentiated by the cytokines characteristically seen in these disorders.

Kawasaki's Disease and Behçet's Disease

Antibodies to endothelial cells are also seen in SLE and Kawasaki's disease, an autoimmune disorder that usually occurs in children. Kawasaki's disease is characterized by arteritis involving large, medium-sized, and small arteries. Coronary arteries and veins are often involved and lymph node involvement is a frequent finding.

Giant cell (temporal) arteritis is the most common type of vasculitis. It's characterized by inflammation of medium and small arteries, primarily the cranial vessels of the brain and the ophthalmic arteries of the eyes. Lesions may be also found in other arteries. Temporal arteritis may be insidious, with a vague onset accompanied by headache, tenderness or severe throbbing pain over the artery.

Visual disturbances, facial pain, and redness and swelling over the overlying skin may also occur. Approximately 50 percent of patients also have systemic involvement and symptoms of polymyalgia rheumatica, a flu-like syndrome characterized by joint symptoms. Visual symptoms vary from blurred or double vision to the sudden onset of blindness that occurs in 40 percent of patients.[21]

Behçet's Disease, which is characterized by painful oral, genital and ocular ulcers, may also cause vasculitis. An autoimmune disorder linked to the HLA antigen DRw52, Behçet's disease may also cause ulceration of the colon and esophagus.

Conventional
Treatment Options

Traditional treatment options focus on reducing inflammation, suppressing the immune system, alleviating pain and correcting hormonal imbalances. In autoimmune blood disorders, treatment involves replacing deficient levels of blood cells and platelets.

New specific therapies, such as monoclonal antibodies and biologics, are geared toward disease prevention as well as symptom relief in that they're designed to manipulate the autoimmune response causing the disease symptoms. This chapter focuses on current options used for the treatment of autoimmune disease.

PRIMARY THERAPIES

Certain primary therapies are used as the mainstay, relieving symptoms in many different ADs. For instance, corticosteroids are widely used because of their ability to suppress the immune system. In fact, a response to corticosteroids is used as a diagnostic tool to help confirm that someone has a disease with an autoimmune origin.

ANTI-INFLAMMATORY AGENTS

Steroid Derivatives

Corticosteroids include a wide variety of synthetic steroid derivatives that interfere with the inflammatory mechanism. Commonly used steroids

155

include prednisone (Deltasone), hydrocortisone, methylprednisolone (Medrol) and dexamethasone (Decadron, Hexadrol). Prednisone is known to reduce levels of vitamins C and B6 and the minerals zinc and potassium, making supplements necessary. Long-term effects of high dose steroids include high blood sugar, infections, cataracts, high blood pressure, increased hair growth, fluid retention and damage to the bones and arteries. Effects increase with higher doses and long-term therapy.

Non-Steroidal Anti-inflammatory Drugs (NSAIDs)

Ibuprofen, naproxen and related compounds have the ability to reduce inflammation although not to the extent that steroids are capable of. Although they do not cause the bone loss and other adverse symptoms associated with steroids, many of the NSAIDs may irritate the lining of the gastric mucosa, causing ulcers and gastrointestinal bleeding. This effect is caused by the diminishment of prostaglandin levels seen with NSAIDs.

Sometimes, other medications such as misoprostol (Cytotec) are also given because of their ability to increase prostaglandin secretion, blocking these effects. However, this drug can cause miscarriage.[1] The following preparations are commonly used to reduce inflammation in SLE and related disorders: acetylsalicylic acid (Aspirin), ibuprofen (Motrin, Advil), diclofenac (Voltaren), diflunisal (Dolobid), oxaproxin (Daypro), naproxen sodium (Naprosyn, Aleve), piroxicam (Feldene), nabumetone (Relafen), indomethacin (Indocin), sulindac (Clinoril), ketoprofen (Orudis), and etodolac (Lodine)

Biologicals (Biological Response Modifiers)

Biologicals are compounds that interfere with the immune response. Interferons are a family of naturally occurring cytokines produced by immune system cells in response to viral infections. One of the most widely used, interferon beta-1a (Avonex), is produced by recombinant DNA technology. Interferon beta exerts its biological actions by binding to specific cell receptors. This binding initiates a complex cascade of immune system events that leads to the production of numerous gene products and markers. Biologicals include the following compounds: immune serums and immunoglobulins, vaccines, systemic hemostatics, and recombinants including Interferon compounds.

Enbrel

Etanercept (Enbrel) binds specifically to tumor necrosis factor (TNF) and blocks its interaction with cell surface TNF receptors. TNF occurs as an intermediate product in the inflammatory process seen in rheumatoid arthritis. However, in October 2000, the European Medicines Evaluation Agency urged doctors to exercise caution when prescribing etanercept because of its link to serious blood reactions.[2]

Immunosuppresant Drugs

Immunosuppressive medications, including immunosuppressive metabolites such as azathioprine, reduce the immune response. Potentially serious toxic effects may result from these medications, primarily alterations in white blood cells due to bone marrow suppression, which may result in infection. Other side effects include bladder problems, hair loss, vomiting, nausea, and fertility problems. Immunosuppressants include: azathioprine (Imuran), cyclosporine (Neoral), methotrexate (Folex, Mexate, Rheumatrex), and mycophenolate mofetil (Cell Cept).

Immunomodulators

Immunomodulators are able to modify immune function. Lefunomide, for instance, can reduce cell proliferation by inhibiting the synthesis of certain amino acids necessary for cell growth. These include glatiramer acetate (Copaxone), lefunonamide (Arava), and thalomid.

Anti-Malarial Drugs

Anti-malarial compounds have been used for many years to treat the joint pain that occurs in rheumatoid arthritis and other connective tissue disorders. Anti-malarials are particularly effective in treating the skin and joint symptoms that occur in SLE and they've proven beneficial in reducing inflammation in many other disorders. These compounds are thought to suppress certain steps in the immune response. Since some medications in this category may have adverse effects on the eyes, regular exams are indicated for patients using anti-malarial drugs. Anti-malarials include: chloroquine (Aralen), hydroxychloroquine (Plaquenil), and quinacrine (Atrabine).

Chemotherapeutic Agents

Chemotherapeutic agents are used both for pain relief and for their immune suppressing properties. Commonly used chemotherapeutic agents include: cyclophosphamide, Methotrexate, and mitoxantrone (Novantrone).

While cyclophosphamide and methotrexate have long been used in autoimmune diseases, including Crohn's disease and scleroderma, mitoxantrone received FDA approval for the treatment of MS in October 2000. The drug was approved for use in patients with the secondary progressive form of MS. Patients using this drug should be carefully monitored for heart problems, a risk that increases with cumulative doses.[3]

MISCELLANEOUS DRUGS USED FOR PAIN RELIEF

Analgesics

Analgesics reduce pain by numbing sensations, although they have no effect on inflammation. Commonly used analgesics include acetaminophen (Tylenol), propoxyphene hydrochloride (Darvon), and narcotics such as oxycodone (Percocet), meperidine hydrochloride (Demerol), morphine sulfate and hydrocodone (Vicodin).

Anticonvulsants

The anticonvulsant medications carbamazepine (Tegretol) and phenytoin (diphenylhydantoin, Dilantin) are often prescribed to relieve facial pain. However, there have been reports of Tegretol increasing MS symptoms.

Tricyclic Antidepressants

Other drugs shown to be effective include the tricyclic antidepressant amitriptyline (Elavil) and gabapentin (Neurontin).

Muscle Relaxants

Baclofen (Lioresal) and tizanidine (Zanaflex) are often used to relieve painful muscle spasms and stiffness.

Intravenous Immunoglobulins

Intravenous immune globulin (IV Ig) therapy (Gammagard, Gammar, Gamine) benefits patients with a number of different ADs. Immune globulins, especially those of class G (IgG globulins), are protein molecules that the body uses to produce antibodies, including autoantibodies. Without sufficient globulin stores, as is seen in several different immune deficiency disorders, the immune system is unable to produce antibodies and fight disease. In ADs, the body's globulin stores are sufficient, but the immune system is defective in that it produces autoantibodies.

Intravenous immunoglobulins (IV Ig) are derived from the plasma of healthy donors. Thus, the autoantibodies, cytokines and other harmful substances in the plasma of patients receiving this therapy are diluted out with healthy immune globulins. In this mode of therapy the immune globulins are introduced directly into the circulation by intravenous transfusion.

IV Ig is particularly valuable in ADs that are mediated or perpetuated by autoantibodies or by immune complex deposits. Immune complexes are formed when antigen and antibodies bind together or when antibodies bind with immune system chemicals known as complement. The presence of immune complexes is generally a poor prognostic sign.

IV Ig Applications

IV Ig therapy is primarily used for treating ADs with a neurologic component, such as demyelinating neuropathies, including multiple sclerosis, multifocal motor neuropathy, inflammatory myopathies, myasthenia gravis, Lambert-Eaton syndrome and pretibial myxedema, a dermatological disorder associated with Graves' disease.

The efficacy of IV Ig has only formally been demonstrated for Guillain-Barré syndrome and the chronic inflammatory polyneuropathies, but favorable reports continue to appear in the literature. For instance, there have been recent reports of a favorable response using this therapy for intractable childhood seizures (Rasmussen's encephalitis).

The basis for using IV Ig lies in its ability to increase the levels of normal globulin present in the blood. As long ago as 1964, researchers observed that the plasma concentration of IgG determined the rate at which these proteins are broken down in the body. All proteins eventually break down, but the rates can be altered. By increasing the body's levels of IgG with immune globulin therapy, the globulin-derived auto-antibodies break down or disintegrate at an accelerated rate. Since it is these autoantibodies that are responsible for most AD symptoms, their removal and reduction in number brings a temporary alleviation of symptoms.

However, the exact mode of action of IV Ig is uncertain. A number of theories have been proposed, but none of them explain all clinical situations. Most likely there are a number of different benefits. For example, it's been demonstrated that high concentrations of immune globulins in plasma, the liquid portion of blood, appear to block the binding ability of autoantibodies. Another explanation is the modulating effect immune globulins have on the immune system. By modulating the immune system, autoantibody production is inhibited. High levels of IgG also affect the response of tissue receptors that are normally affected by autoantibodies. Saturated with immunoglobulin, receptors in skin, muscle, and intestinal epithelium are less likely to respond to the untoward effects of autoantibodies.

Precautions

There have been several reports of both acute myocardial infarction and vascular complications occurring during or soon after treatment with high dose intravenous immunoglobulins.[4]

MONOCLONAL ANTIBODY THERAPY

Monoclonal antibodies designed with specific body proteins can modify the immune response. Examples include the drug infliximab (Remicade) used in Crohn's disease and rheumatoid arthritis (RA) and rituximab (Rituxan). Expression of the cytokine known as tumor necrosis factor-α (TNF-α) is increased in Crohn's disease. Another cytokine known as nuclear factor kappa-β controls the inflammatory response, including expression of necrosis factor-α. Monoclonal antibody therapy (prescription medication Infliximab) directed against TNF-α results in a remission rate of 30 percent to 50 percent after 4 weeks, although it is primarily used for patients who show no response to conventional therapy.

Monoclonal antibodies are protein substances that have a single, selected specificity making them seek out and latch onto a specific cell type. Monoclonal antibodies are continuously secreted and thereby produced by "immortalized" hybridoma cells. A hybridoma is a biologically constructed hybrid of a mortal, antibody producing lymphoid cell and a malignant or immortal myeloma cell.

In patients with RA, the combination of infliximab and methotrexate offers dramatic results. Infliximab is the first FDA approved drug touted to prevent the worsening of symptoms and inhibit the production of structural damage.[5]

Use in MS

Researchers at Mayo Clinic have proven that damaged myelin can be repaired with monoclonal antibodies. In this therapy, the antibodies, which were derived from patients with monoclonal gammopathies, were able to bind to damaged oligodendrocytes (the central nervous system support cells which are damaged in demyelinating diseases) in vitro. This therapy is currently being tested in clinical trials.[6]

TREATMENT OF
VASCULAR DISEASES, NEUROPATHIES

Treatment for these conditions focuses on correcting the hypertension and clotting problems associated with these disorders. Antihypertensive agents are the mainstay and include both beta adrenergic blocking agents and calcium channel blockers. Procardia, in particular, is useful for reducing blood pressure and alleviating symptoms of Raynaud's phenomenon and vasculitis.

DRUGS USED TO CORRECT
CHEMICAL IMBALANCES AND ANEMIA

Hormones

In patients with hormone deficiencies, standard hormonal preparations such as glucocorticoid steroids, thyroid hormone, and insulin are routinely prescribed.

Blood Components

Red blood cells are used to treat the anemia seen in many ADs. The liquid or plasma portion of blood, when frozen and thawed before use, contains clotting factors essential for patients with deep vein thrombosis and other symptoms of an impaired clotting mechanism such as antiphospholipid syndrome. Platelets, blood components essential for clotting, are reduced in autoimmune thrombocytopenic purpura and from the administration of many different drugs. Platelet transfusions are routinely ordered to correct critical platelet deficiencies.

SPECIFIC AUTOIMMUNE
DISEASE THERAPIES

Pemphigus and Myasthenia Gravis

In autoimmune pemphigus, systemic glucocorticosteroid treatment is life-saving, but it may cause severe side effects. However, similar to the disease mechanism in myasthenia gravis, alterations in acetylcholine also play a role in pemphigus disease development, making acetylcholine inhibitors a primary treatment modality.

Mestinon (pyridostigmine bromide)

Mestinon inhibits the destruction of acetylcholine by the enzyme acetylcholinesterase and thereby permits stronger adhesion of the keratinocyte skin cells. Acetylcholine competes with the destructive pemphigus antibodies, preventing them from attaching to keratinocytes. The destructive antibodies are both autoantibodies to keratinocyte acetylcholine receptors (seen in 85 percent of pemphigus patients and most patients with MG) and autoantibodies to the adhesion molecules desmoglein 1 and 3.

Mestinon is FDA approved for the muscle weakness of myasthenia gravis but it's experimental for pemphigus patients. Clinical trials are currently being held to assess the efficacy of mestinon at University of California–Davis Medical Center in Sacramento (for information contact sagrando@ucdavis.edu).[7]

Graves' Disease

In autoimmune hyperthyroidism or Graves' disease, levels of thyroid hormone are too high. Therapy aims to reduce thyroid hormone levels in the blood by limiting the amount of thyroid tissue capable of producing hormone via surgery or radioiodine ablation, or by reducing the body's supply of iodine with anti-thyroid drugs or alternative medicine.

Multiple Sclerosis

A variety of new drugs and treatment protocols have been recently designed to reduce symptoms in MS, including the following.

Glatirimer acetate, Copolymer 1 (Copaxone)

Glatiramer acetate, an approved therapy for MS, is a polymer comprising a random sequence of 4 amino acids (L-alanine, L-glutamine, L-tyrosine, and L-lysine) initially designed to mimic the activity of myelin basic protein. Glatiramer has been found to reduce lymphocyte proliferation by perhaps acting as a superantigen capable of inducing anergy or death of potentially pathogenic cells.[8] The mechanism of action of glatiramer may include the induction of Th2 cytokines to multiple myelin antigens.

Novantrone

Novantrone, manufactured by Immunex Corporation, is used to slow the worsening of neurologic disability and to reduce the relapse rate in patients with clinically worsening forms of relapsing-remitting and secondary progressive multiple sclerosis. Clinical trial results demonstrated that Novantrone had a statistically significant impact on reduction of relapse rate and delay in disability progression. There was a 65 percent reduction in annual relapse rate compared to placebo and a 64 percent reduction in 1-point Expanded Disability Status Scale (EDSS) deterioration confirmed at six months. Novantrone works by suppressing the activity of T cells, B cells and macrophages that are thought to lead the attack on the myelin sheet. Side effects include nausea, hair loss, upper respiratory tract infections, and transient neutropenia.[9]

Interferon-β and Interferon-γ

Interferon-β and Interferon-γ represent the yin and yang of immunomodulation in MS. The gamma (γ) form of interferon is a potent inflammatory mediator and an activator of the disease activity in MS because it upregulates MHC class II expression on helper T cells and macrophages. These are the two major components of the inflammatory lesion in the brain of MS patients.

Administration of IFN-γ induces MHC class II expression on microglial and astrocytes cells in the central nervous system, allowing them to act as antigen presenting cells to T cells. Clinical trials showed improvement in some patients while others experienced increased disease activity.

Interferon-β is an immunomodulator with many activities that oppose IFN-γ. For instance, it inhibits the synthesis of IFN-γ produced by T lymphocytes and downregulates MHC class II expression on antigen presenting cells. In clinical trials, IFN-β was shown to favorably alter the natural course of MS. Slowing of disease progression and decrease in activity on MR scans was noted. However, IFN-β may trigger the development of other autoimmune disorders.

Thalamic Stimulation

Thalamic stimulation is surgically achieved through use of a deep brain stimulation system. Preoperative and postoperative symptoms are routinely assessed so that benefits can be weighed. Thalamic stimulation has been proven to be effective in reducing tremor associated with MS. However, other MS symptoms, such as memory impairment, do not benefit from this process, and in some instances, visuospatial coordination worsened after thalamic stimulation surgery.

Autoimmune Hemolytic Anemia

Plasma Exchange

In plasma exchange, patients are transfused with large amounts, usually two to three liters, of compatible fresh plasma for 5 to 7 consecutive days. Although plasma exchanges succeed in diluting autoantibodies, the effects are generally short lived since autoantibodies are constantly being produced.

Blood Transfusions

If anemia is severe, transfusions of packed red blood cells may be indicated. However, crossmatching blood for patients with autoimmune hemolytic anemia may be a diagnostic challenge. Erythrocyte (red blood cell) autoantibodies may interfere with methods used to detect alloantibodies for other blood group antigens. Furthermore, up to 50 percent of transfused red blood cells may be destroyed by the patient's red cell antibodies. A blood warmer is recommended by the American Association of Blood Banks for transfusing patients who have cold reacting red cell antibodies.

Immunosuppressants

Corticosteroids, which inhibit antibody production as well as the release of lysosomal enzymes, are also used as a primary therapy in autoimmune hemolytic anemia. Patients with marked hemolysis may require intravenous steroids administered at high doses. Other immunosuppressive drugs such as cyclophosphamide may also be used, and IV Igs may also be used in an attempt to halt the body's own autoantibody production.

Several reports indicate that cyclosporine-A used in conjunction with steroids during the early stages of the disease allowed patients the opportunity to use less steroids. The use of cyclosporine-A is reported to represent a useful corticosteroid sparer in the maintenance of clinical remission in patients with early-stage, active SLE.

Lupus Nephritis

Treatment for lupus nephritis generally depends on the severity of the disease. Recent treatment advances in this area have led to higher life expectancy for patients with renal complications of lupus. Patients with lupus nephritis usually have more than one type of lesion, such as membranous or mesangial nephropathy. Patients with a mesangial proliferative glomerulonephritis or membranous nephropathy usually respond to oral prednisolone, occasionally with the addition of azathioprine as a steroid sparing agent.

Patients with a severe proliferative or narcotizing glomerulonephritis or with extracapillary proliferation benefit from the addition of cyclophosphamide. A study conducted by the NIH showed that oral prednisolone together with monthly intravenous pulses of cyclophosphamide for six months, followed by quarterly pulses for an additional two years, was more effective than monthly pulses of prednisolone alone.[10]

Primary Biliary Cirrhosis (PBC)

Long-term administration of ursodeoxycholic acid (UDCA) has been found to be both safe and effective for reducing symptoms of PBC. By stimulating bile flow, UDCA slows bile duct destruction and fibrosis and delays the onset of cirrhosis. In patients who don't respond well to UDCA, combined therapy with corticosteroids appears to be more promising. Studies using UDCA in combination with colcicine or methotrexate showed no additional benefits. The primary reason for not responding to UDCA therapy is that autoimmune hepatitis is also present, with symptoms of both diseases overlapping. This explains why a favorable response is seen when corticosteroids are administered along with UDCA. For patients entering the terminal stage of PBC, liver transplantation remains the only therapeutic option.

Systemic Lupus Erythematosus

Administered at 200 mg/day in clinical trials, treatment resulted in improved objective and subjective measurements of disease activity. Since many SLE patients have low DHEA levels, which appear to be even lower in patients also receiving steroids, patients in the trials achieved supra-physiologic levels of DHEA and a relative increase in testosterone compared to estrogen. The main improvement noted was relief of myalgia and fatigue.[11]

Mycophenolic acid mofetil (1.5–2 g/day) was reported to be useful in lupus patients with renal disease.[12]

Raynaud's Syndrome

L-arginine or sodium nitroprusside, used to increase the blood concentration of nitric oxide, has been reported to block symptoms in Raynaud's attacks suffered by patients with scleroderma. Related research studies are being conducted at Wayne State University's behavioral medicine laboratory. For more information, call 313-577-1889.

Estrogen has long been suspected of triggering Raynaud's. Postmenopausal women who take estrogen alone are reported to suffer more from Raynaud's phenomenon than women who either don't take estrogen or take a combination of hormones.

Calcium channel blockers are used to relax and dilate blood vessels. The two most common therapies include Procardia and Nifedipine. Prescription nitroglycerin ointment offers relief when applied directly to the affected digits, and it can be used as a preventive or defensive therapy.

Psoriasis

Laser Photonics, Inc., has received FDA approval to use their excimer laser system for treatment of psoriasis. Unlike the ultraviolet phototherapy treatments traditionally used, excimer laser treatment can be given at the high doses needed for rapid clearing. The excimer laser system delivers ultraviolet light directly to psoriasis plaques via fiber optics, reducing the cancer risk to non-affected skin.

Alternative Medical Treatment Options

Like an excitable puppy, the immune system is influenced by many divergent factors. A harsh tone influences the disposition of both the puppy and one's immune system cells. Other influences include diet, temperature, injuries, toxins, age, time, boredom, loneliness, and even the stress of wondering where the next meal is coming from.

Although the negative effects on immunity caused by suffering, stress and pain have been known since Hans Selye's initial studies in the 1930s, it's only been in recent years that researchers have discovered the positive effects of stress reduction. Previously, a positive response to stress reduction, such as that experienced by Dr. Norman Cousins, was considered merely anecdotal. After all, in 1950, there were no scientific methods available to measure cytokine levels or changes in neuroendocrine cells.

Since the 1980s, many studies have demonstrated that both diet and stress reduction techniques directly influence the immune system's key players, the lymphocytes and cytokines. In this chapter I describe the role of alternative medicine in treating ADs. While space prohibits an extensive exploration of all therapies, this chapter offers broad insight into the value of self-care in healing ADs.

EMOTIONS AND HEALTH

In March 2001, medical experts gathered at the National Institutes of Health to discuss what only a decade ago would have been considered new age fluff. These experts discussed the mind-body connection, affirming the notion that molecular changes in the nervous system have a direct bearing on immune function and health.

DIET

Diet is a well-known mediator of immune system function. What one eats can stimulate, weaken, balance or strengthen the immune system. Foods that balance and strengthen the immune system are desirable for autoimmune diseases, while foods that weaken or stimulate the immune system are to be avoided. Furthermore, certain immune influences are associated with specific foods. For instance, animal studies have shown that a diet high in alfalfa may cause blood changes similar to what is seen in patients with lupus. It's suspected that the amino acid L-canavanine in alfalfa is responsible.

Saturated Fats

Many studies indicate that antioxidants in fresh fruits and vegetables offer the greatest benefits for ADs while saturated fats, refined sugar and caffeine cause the most detrimental effects. Diets high in saturated fat have been found to produce disturbances in lymphocyte functioning. In one study animals fed high fat diets were prone to developing lupus. However, when the animals were switched to a low fat diet, kidney inflammation and autoantibody levels diminished. And in Japan, women who frequently eat fatty meats, such as beef and pork, are reported to have a higher risk for developing SLE.

High fat diets are also associated with the development of MS. Cholesterol and high levels of saturated fats in the American diet lead to the production of prostaglandin-2, a hormone-like substance that stimulates the inflammatory response and intensifies negative MS symptoms. Some researchers suggest that people with MS consume less than15 grams of saturated fat/day.[1] The following sections describe the immune system effects of specific food components.

Antioxidants

Antioxidants are chemicals that neutralize free radical molecules. Free radicals are naturally occurring oxygen molecules that play a significant role in the aging process and are responsible for much of the inflammation characteristic of autoimmune diseases. Some of the richest sources of antioxidants include teas, herbs, and most fruits and vegetables. The antioxidant herb *Silymarin* or milk thistle is well known for protecting the liver against environmental toxins and for helping restore the integrity of liver cells. Several reports indicate that antioxidant levels are typically low in people with ADs.

For the past decade, researchers have focused their efforts on the antioxidants found in berries and cherries. Scientists at the University of Texas Health Science Center at Antonio recently identified the antioxidant melatonin in cherries, and researchers at the University of Michigan have found bioflavinoids and acanthocyanins. These antioxidants are reported to be ten times more active than vitamin C.

Bioflavinoids and Acanthocyanins

Bioflavinoids, including phytoestrogen compounds, are natural chemical antioxidants found in plants that have the potential to inhibit the enzymes cyclooxygenase-1 and 2 (COX-1 and COX-2). Inhibiting these enzymes prevents and reduces inflammation in the body. Foods naturally high in bioflavinoids include berries, cherries and grapes and herbs such as catnip and other mints. The scientist Albert Szent-Gyogyi originally discovered bioflavinoids in 1928, although he called them vitamin P.

Acanthocyanins comprise a group of antioxidant chemicals responsible for the bright color seen in berries and cherries. Recently, researchers at Michigan State University identified three powerful acanthocyanins in tart cherries. These particular acanthocyanins have the potential to inhibit the growth of colon cancer and they're known to inhibit cyclooxygenase 1 and 2. Twenty cherries provide 25 milligrams of acanthocyanins, an amount sufficient to inhibit the enzymes that cause tissue inflammation and pain.

Acanthocyanins may also protect artery walls from the damage that leads to plaque formation.[2] Amway Corporation of Grand Rapids, Michigan, recently licensed the patent from Michigan State University and is conducting clinical trials on the role of tart cherries in reducing inflammation.

Nutrient Deficiencies and Dietary Supplements

Essential fatty acids

A number of ADs, including autoimmune thyroid disorders and MS, are associated with essential fatty acid deficiencies. Benefits are seen with the addition of evening primrose and flaxseed oils. And in some ADs, such as RA and IBS, omega 3 fatty acids found in fish appear to offer a protective effect. Essential fatty acids should always be added slowly because some fatty acids, including those found in vegetable oils, may cause inflammation, worsening symptoms in some ADs.

Vitamin D

Certain ADs, including Graves' disease, multiple sclorosis, celiac disease and IBS, are associated with vitamin D_3 deficiencies. The increased metabolism in GD and the malabsorption commonly seen in IBS and celiac disease inhibit the absorption of oil soluble vitamins. As with essential oils, oil soluble vitamins should be added slowly and supplemental doses should not exceed 600 International Units daily unless prescribed by one's physician. Excess vitamin D can cause nausea, weakness, constipation and irritability.

People with superior vitamin D status, such as those living in higher altitudes, are known to have milder autoimmune disease symptoms and a lower rate of autoimmune disorders. Adequate vitamin D causes the parathyroid glands to secrete less parathyroid hormone. One of the causes of autoimmune disease is the failure of thymocyte cells in the thymus to destroy T cells destined to become autoreactive. Thymocytes do this by ordering the apoptosis or programmed cell death of autoreactive cells. According to current theory, parathyroid hormone may inhibit apoptosis in thymocytes.[3]

Vitamin E

Vitamin E is a potent antioxidant particularly helpful in malabsorption disorders such as celiac disease. By quenching free radicals, vitamin E may also prevent some of the nervous system and other damage caused by insulin dependent diabetes mellitus. Daily supplements of 800–900 International Units are generally safe, although people who are taking blood thinners or who are deficient in vitamin K should not take vitamin E. However, patients taking anticonvulsants, cholesterol-lowering drugs, tuberculosis drugs, ulcer medication or neomycin generally require higher doses of vitamin E. In fact, the worsening of symptoms seen in MS patients using the anticonvulsant carbamazepine may be caused by vitamin E deficiencies.

It's also important that vitamins are balanced properly since imbalances can aggravate symptoms in some autoimmune disorders. While vitamin E supplements can benefit scleroderma, polymyositis and lupus, cigarette smoke can deplete vitamins C and E, causing imbalances in lupus patients who are taking vitamin E alone.[4]

Vitamin A

A recent study conducted at Penn State University suggests that vitamin A's active form may enhance the effectiveness of interferon. The reason behind this study was the realization that vitamin A deficiency affects inflammation as well as the immune response. In the Penn State experiment, human macrophage cells were stimulated under both vitamin A deficient and sufficient conditions. Enhanced activity of interferon was noted in both conditions with the addition of vitamin A.[5]

Dietary Foes and Friends

To autoimmune disease researchers, it's no surprise that autoimmune diseases are rarely seen in undeveloped countries. Studies of Saharan black Africans indicate that the traditional quasi-vegetarian diets of this population offers them protection. The increased vitamin D levels of this population also have a protective effect.

While there are many reports of low fat, vegetarian diets reducing symptoms in autoimmune diseases, alfalfa should be avoided as it has been found to cause lupus-like symptoms. And foods from the nightshade family, such as eggplants, peppers, and tomatoes, can cause inflammation in susceptible individuals, especially those with rheumatoid arthritis because they contain solanine, which increases pain and swelling.

Essential fatty acids provided by oily fish and flaxseed oil are beneficial for patients with many autoimmune diseases, including SLE, MS and autoimmune thyroid disorders. Bromelain, found in fresh pineapple, and vitamin B complex both help reduce inflammation.

Prednisone therapy can cause deficiencies in vitamins C, B6 and potassium. Patients with SLE should avoid taking iron supplements because they may increase pain, inflammation and joint destruction.[6]

Specific Disease Dietary Recommendations

Chronic Fatigue Syndrome

Patients with chronic fatigue generally benefit from antioxidants such as vitamin A (maximum dose 15,000 IU daily), 800 IU of vitamin E, 1,000–3,000 mg of vitamin C, 100 mg of vitamin B complex and 50 mg of zinc. Sixty mg of Coenzyme Q 10 should also be added to boost circulation, and a complex of 2,000 mg calcium and 1,000 mg of magnesium helps decrease pain and improve muscle function. Also, 1,000 mg of the amino acid L-Glutamine helps improve mental function. A complex of magnesium-potassium aspartate can also be used to increase energy levels.[7]

Fibromyalgia

An optimal diet for patients with fibromyalgia includes whole foods, including vegetables, fruits, nuts, seeds, whole grains and lean poultry. Patients with fibromyalgia should avoid foods high in fat (increases inflammation) and minimize consumption of sugar, caffeine and alcohol because they increase fatigue and pain. Digestive enzymes are often used to aid digestion and nutrient absorption. The supplements used for chronic fatigue syndrome have also proven beneficial. Acidophilus tablets should also be taken to impede the growth of yeast, a common occurrence in patients with fibromyalgia.

Pulsed signal therapy (PST), which shows great potential for fibromyalgia and arthritis, works on painful, inflamed joints, especially those linked to the neck and back. PST, which works through magnetic fields, sends signals directly to connective tissue and cartilage and boosts the body's self-healing properties. Although this treatment is approved in Europe, FDA approval is still pending in Mexico and the United States.

Multiple Sclerosis

Choline (1,000 mg taken twice daily) is thought to protect the myelin sheath from damage. Patients with MS are often deficient in vitamin B_{12} so often B_{12} injections are used therapeutically.

A number of patients have reported achieving remission from MS by following dietary changes and adding supplements. In a recent Life Extension patient profile, one patient describes her successful regimen, which included DHEA, progesterone, pregnenolone, digestive enzymes, antioxidants, and a phyoto-herbal mix consisting of assorted amino acids, herbs, minerals, vitamins, and essential fatty acids.[8]

Systemic Lupus Erythematosus and Rheumatoid Arthritis

Patients with both SLE and RA benefit from dietary or supplemental sulfur. Sulfur helps repair and rebuild connective tissue, cartilage and bone and helps with the absorption of calcium. Sulfur is found in garlic, onions, eggs and asparagus and in various commercial supplements, including MSM.

Essential fatty acids and glucosamine sulfate supplements have also proven beneficial as have the antioxidants listed in the section on chronic fatigue syndrome.

IMMUNOMODULATORS

Immunomodulators are natural substances or synthetic preparations that promote immune system balance. Immunomodulators include plant sterols and sterolins, Reishi Mushroom Extract, German Chamomile, and flower pollen extracts such as Cernitin and Prostaphil. Plant sterols are available commercially in 20 mg capsules of Sterinol, which is taken 3 times daily, and in products made from the Polynesian plant *Morinda citrifolia* such as Noni, Nonu, and Nono.

BEHAVIORAL MODIFICATION

Biofeedback

According to researchers at Johns Hopkins University, biofeedback can be used with success to control blood flow in patients with Raynaud's phenomenon.[9] And biofeedback, a form of behavior modification that alters our usual response to certain factors, is what Dr. Norman Cousins used to achieve remission from his own ankylosing spondylitis.

NATURAL ELEMENTS

In traditional Chinese Medicine, disease development is linked to seasonal variations, including climate and temperature. These are taken into consideration in prescribing therapy. Similarly, in allopathic medicine it's known that sunlight can exacerbate SLE, and heat can aggravate MS. While people with fibromyalgia benefit from moist heat, recent studies indicate that alternating periods of heat and cold can be effective. However, drafty, cool areas can trigger muscle spasms and pain.[10]

FOOD ALLERGIES

Food allergies have long been associated with autoimmune diseases. Numerous studies have shown increased levels of IgE (associated with allergy) in patients with AITD, SLE and MS. Furthermore, the immune system is compromised when challenged by allergens, exacerbating AD symptoms.

HERBAL THERAPY

Herbal therapy is used for many autoimmune disorders, particularly SLE. Herbs used in lupus include red clover, echinacea (used intermittently in periods not to exceed six weeks), feverfew and pau d'arco. *Lycopus virginicus* (bugleweed) and *Melissa officianalis* (lemon balm) have been reported by the German Commission E to be safe and efficacious for reducing thyroid hormone levels in patients with Graves' disease. And gotu kola has been reported to improve symptoms in scleroderma.

However, herbal therapy can have serious complications. For this reason, it's essential that patients report herbal usage to their physician. While the toxicity of some herbs is well known, the effects of herbs on other drugs haven't been fully studied. Herbs known to cause liver damage include borage, coltsfoot, jin bu huan, margosa oil, mistletoe, sassafrass and skullcap. Herbs that can damage the kidneys include calamus, chapparal, germander, and germanium. Herbs associated with veno-occlusive disease, heart failure or hypertension include comfrey, ephedra, and licorice root. Before adding any herbs, patients should check with the

NIH Office of Dietary Supplements or The American Botanical Council (see resource chapter).

HORMONE THERAPY

Various hormones have been tested for their autoimmune influences. Overall, estrogens promote autoimmune disease development, while testosterone and progesterone have been found to provide a protective effect.

Melatonin, although it is effective in promoting sleep, is not recommended for patients with certain autoimmune disorders, including rheumatoid arthritis and lupus.[11]

A number of studies have shown that many patients with autoimmune disease are deficient in DHEA (see chapter 8), growth hormone (GH) and somatomedin C, a hormone involved in muscle repair. GH deficiency also adds to aches and pains because it has a role in removing lactic acid and other byproducts of muscle metabolism. Because hormone imbalances vary among the many autoimmune disorders, glandular and hormonal supplements, even homeopathic preparations, should only taken under medical supervision.

EXERCISE

Taoist Tai Chi

Patients with AD may wish to check out the Taoist Tai Chi Society (TTCS). There are many different styles of tai chi, but this particular form is devoted entirely to improving health. The TTCS also has a "special needs" group for people with arthritis, MS, MD, AIDS, cancer, osteoporosis, ankylosing spondylitis, Parkinson's disease, and other degenerative disorders. Many patients with these disorders have reduced or eliminated their need for medication from regularly practicing tai chi. It's not a magic pill; it doesn't work unless you practice it regularly, but there are accounts of people who literally abandoned their wheelchairs after following this program.

Yoga

For many years, people have used Yoga as an exercise discipline that incidentally promotes healing. The deep breathing exercises and cleansing breaths are thought to improve immune system functioning.

STRESS REDUCTION

Stress directly contributes to AD development. People with ADs and people who are chronically stressed or depressed are known to have low cytokine levels. In stress, macrophages are unable to produce the cytokines interleukin-2, interleukin-1 and tumor necrosis factor. Stress also interferes with the production of cytokines such as interferon.

Dr. Joan Borysenko, describing the consequences of stress in *The Power of the Mind to Heal, Renewing Body, Mind, and Spirit*, reports that even temporary stress can completely wipe out the body's interferon levels. Without interferon, NK cells can't do their jobs of destroying autoreactive lymphocytes. Furthermore, subjected to chronic stress, the body prepares to die. This is evidenced by changes in the body's levels of neuropeptides, enkephalins, and endorphins designed to make us sleepy and numb.

Borysenko, a psychologist and a pioneer in the field of psychoneuroimmunology at Harvard University, describes the importance of cultivating a social network of family and friends. Joy, she says, elicits a positive response in each of the body's cells. Diet has a similar influence because food molecules affect the immune cells lining our guts. These cells, in turn, release neuropeptides that affect our emotions. And our emotions go on to affect our immune system health. Besides the necessity of a nutrient rich diet and a social network, the immune system also responds favorably to touch.

As a vivid example, Borysenko describes an experiment in which rabbits were given chemicals known to cause atherosclerotic lesions and heart disease. Rabbits in the lower level of cages, however, remained immune to the effects of these chemicals. The experiment was considered flawed and had to be repeated. The results were the same. An investigation showed that the technician managing the experiment always patted the rabbits in the lower berth, but she couldn't reach those in the higher cages.[12]

Not Enough Stress

It's long been established that the effects of stress are cumulative, and it's our response to stress, not stress itself, that causes problems. Over time, chronic stress causes an allostatic load, which disrupts the normal stress response. Bruce McEwen, a neuroscientist at Rockefeller University, explains that inadequate production of stress hormones can be just as harmful as too much. A diminished response to stress, such as seen in apathy, may trigger the secretion of other substances that compensate for the loss. For example, if cortisol doesn't increase in response to stress, inflammatory cytokines, which are regulated by cortisol, will rise.[13]

THE USE OF CANNABINOIDS IN MS

For many years, the medicinal benefits of cannabinoids (marijuana) have been studied. In one recent study, cannabinoids were found to be effective in controlling the tremors and muscle spasticity experienced by MS patients. In the study, mice with experimental allergic encephalomyelitis, a condition with symptoms similar to that seen in MS, were given synthetic cannabinoid compounds. The compounds were found to stimulate cannabinoid receptors on the surface of nerve cells.[14]

ENERGY HEALING

Energy healing includes a number of different therapies designed to restore balance to the body's natural healing system or life force. In some therapies, the goal is to restore or replenish yin or yang, depending on the particular symptoms and the patient's individual constitution. Therapies commonly employed include acupuncture, moxibustion, jin shen do, bright light therapy, music therapy and acupressure.

Current Research Trends

It's nearly as impossible to list all the triggers of AD as it is to list all the ADs. Difficulty in listing the triggers arises because ADs are not acute disorders. They develop slowly. Often, years pass from the beginning of symptoms to the time of diagnosis. Furthermore, even when the cause seems obvious, as is the case with occupational exposure to silica and scleroderma, the reports are anecdotal at best.

To establish definite causes using peer-reviewed studies, researchers would have to expose human beings to the suspected triggers, many of which are toxic, and observe these individuals for immune system changes. Obviously, such an experiment is out of the question. Even in a more humane context involving direct testing of chemicals, we find that environmental chemicals are rarely tested for their immune system effects. In the event that the Environmental Protection Agency decides such studies are needed, the burden of proof generally lies with the chemical industry. And unfortunately, only a small number of chemicals are deemed worthy of such studies.

Even then, such studies become weapons, with the manufacturing company often financing university studies and suggesting what the desirable outcome should be. And as Sheldon Krimsky points out in *Hormonal Chaos*, the chemical manufacturing industry has their own army of scientists ready to contest any unfavorable studies. In reviewing the controversy surrounding endocrine disruptors in the following section, we're afforded insight into how public policy is influenced and how policy often works against us.

Xenobiotics

Xenobiotics refer to environmental substances that have biologic effects on humans. However, studies of xenobiotics generally fail to consider that fetuses might be more sensitive to exposure to xenobiotics than newborns or young children. Krimsky explains that detoxification mechanisms do not develop until after birth. Young children have fat deposits where xenobiotics are stored. Fetuses lack this buffer and they do not yet have the blood brain barrier that normally protects brain cells from toxic substances. And one of the targets of endocrine disrupting chemicals is the immune system.[1]

DEVELOPMENTAL EFFECTS

In 1996, scientists at the Wingspread Conference Center in Racine, Wisconsin, gathered to discuss this problem, later presented in their report, "Chemically Induced Alterations in the Developing Immune System: The Wildlife/Human Connection." In this report, scientists explained how immune system changes in the fetus caused by endocrine disruptors do not generally show up until adulthood, emerging as cancer or ADs.

Even so, many endocrine disrupting chemicals remain in the workplace. The reason may have to do with rewards. According to Dan Fagin, writing in the Center for Public Integrity's 1999 exposé, *Toxic Deception: How the Chemical Industry Manipulates Science, Bends the Law and Endangers Your Health:* "Virtually half of the EPA officials who left top-level jobs in toxics and pesticides during the past 15 years went to work for chemical companies, their trade associations, or their lobbying firms."[2]

SCREENING TESTS FOR
AUTOIMMUNE IMMUNOTOXICITY

Traditionally, the toxicity of chemicals relies on studies designed to assess substances for their propensity to cause cancer or overt birth defects. Toxicity studies do not routinely determine immune enhancing effects. Furthermore, toxicology protocols follow the principle "the dose makes the poison." According to this notion, any substance can be toxic at a high enough dose, and in low doses, any substance is harmless. Another tenet of this canon is that an organism is not adversely affected by doses lower than toxic levels. However, Krimsky has found several studies challenging this view.

For example, at high doses, estrogenic chemicals fed to pregnant mice inhibited the normal development of the prostate in male offspring.

In contrast, doses 10,000 times lower administered to pregnant mice resulted in a permanent increase in the prostate size of the male offspring. Thus, traditional toxicology canons may miss the effects of small doses on the developing organism.[3]

Researchers at the 1999 North Carolina conference linking environmental agents to AD addressed the need for immunotoxicity testing. The consensus was that in standard toxicity testing the adverse immune systems effects of chemicals are often if not always missed. To date, the most promising assay available for determining autoimmune-inducing effects in chemicals is the popliteal lymph node assay.

Popliteal Lymph Node Assay

According to current theory, lymphocytes require two signals to become activated. The first signal is provided by cell receptors upon recognizing a specific antigen. Co-stimulatory molecules and cytokines provide the second signal.

Generally, low molecular weight compounds (LMWCs) are responsible for the first signal. Although they are too small on their own to act as antigen, they may bind to the body's proteins, forming a hapten-carrier complex or they may alter the bound protein molecules. Alternately, LMWCs can influence antigen presentation so that previously cryptic epitopes may be presented by MHC molecules linked to antigen presenting cells.

In both cases, the hapten-carrier complexes or the cryptic epitopes are recognized as new. These compounds elicit the first signal. If these chemicals also cause induction of cytokines, immunostimulation and immunosensitization may follow.[4]

In the popliteal lymph node assay (PLNA), chemicals are injected subcutaneously into the footpad of mice or rats. Six to eight days later, lymph nodes are measured. Enlargement is a sign of immunostimulating potential. In 1999, little more than 100 chemicals were tested by PLNA, which has several procedural variations. In the simplest form, the test fails to distinguish immunostimulating haptens from inflammatory irritants.

OUR CHEMICAL LEGACY

Even when chemicals capable of inducing ADs are identified, the problem often remains. Because many of these chemicals are pervasive and lodge in fat deposits, they're passed from generation to generation. And even when they're banned, other problems occur. For instance, pressures on poor countries to ban the insecticide DDT have led to a resurgence of malaria. Because DDT has been exempted from the Convention on Persistent Organic Pollutants, a legally binding treaty designed to reduce organic pollutant contamination, it will likely be put into use again in poor countries.[5]

Even the problem of thimerosal is unlikely to be resolved soon. While the NIH recommends that pregnant women (weighing on the average 50 kg) refrain from eating more than a can of tuna daily because it has 17 mcg of mercury, two month old infants (weighing about 5 kg) are routinely given vaccines containing 62.5 mcg of mercury.[6]

SUSPECTED AUTOIMMUNE CONDITIONS

The list of autoimmune disorders continues to grow, and the number of disorders suspected of having an autoimmune origin, such as chronic fatigue syndrome and fibromyalgia, also continues to escalate. Often, however, a definitive link is hard to establish. For instance, sensorineural hearing loss has suspected of having ties to immunity since 1958. Since then, a number of studies have shown evidence of this involvement, including a response to steroid therapy. Patients with what appears to be autoimmune sensorineural hearing loss usually present with bilateral progressive hearing loss, and 65 percent of all cases occur in females between the ages of 17 to 42 years.[7]

CLINICAL TRIALS

Clinical trials are used to study the efficacy and safety of drugs and other therapeutic protocols before their formal introduction. The benefits of clinical trials include the opportunity to try new therapies before they're introduced to the public and to aid in scientific research. And on occasion, patients who are initially given placebos in clinical trials are later given the opportunity to become test subjects. See the resource chapter for information on participating in clinical trials.

NIEHS Research Groups

The National Institute of Environmental Health Sciences in Research Triangle Park, North Carolina, continues its assessment of environmental chemicals and their involvement in autoimmune disease development. Currently, a research group is investigating the role of environmental agents in the development of myositis, a chronic, incurable, potentially fatal autoimmune disorder affecting muscles, including heart muscle. This group will later expand to continue its research into the development of other ADs.

TREATMENT NEWS

Antigen Specific Therapy

According to the National Institute of Allergy and Infectious Diseases (NIAID), a new therapy, which is currently being tested on monkeys with a disease similar to multiple sclerosis (MS), could soon be tested against MS and other ADs in humans.

Known as antigen specific immunotherapy, treatment specifically targets the immune system's T cells. Dr. Michael Lenardo of NIAID, who discovered this therapy, found that in MS, T cells that are exposed to small amounts of the proteins making up the myelin sheath are stimulated to attack the sheath.

However, when T cells are exposed to large amounts of these proteins, they undergo a preprogrammed self-destruct sequence. (In fact, T cells exposed to large amounts of any protein will self-destruct.) Thus, introducing large amounts of myelin proteins into the body should, in theory, destroy the problematic T cells in MS, inhibiting the disease process.

And indeed it has, in a number of experimental studies. Using this therapy on monkeys, Dr. Lenardo was able to show, by magnetic resonance imaging studies (MRI), a reduction of the disease process. Furthermore, the treatment appeared to cause no adverse affects. Current studies are focusing on mice with myasthenia gravis.

This therapy has the potential to alleviate symptoms in a number of different ADs. Similar to oral tolerance therapy, a treatment showing promising results in studies of patients with type 1 diabetes, antigen specific immunotherapy shows great promise in bringing relief to those suffering from ADs.

Prolactin

For several years, researchers have studied the role of the hormone prolactin in modulating autoimmune diseases, particularly systemic lupus erythematosus.

Diabetes vaccines

According to a study published in the prestigious journal *Science*, a single protein may stimulate the body's immune system to destroy the pancreatic islet cells that produce insulin. The protein, identified as glutamic acid decarboxylase (GAD), triggered an autoimmune response in mice similar to that seen in humans.[8] Its role as a target self-antigen holds great promise for a preventive vaccine. A vaccine capable of suppressing the genetic expression of GAD may have therapeutic value in IDDM.

In another recent study, vaccines that promote Th2 cells and inhibit Th1 cells have been shown to prevent diabetes development in mice with advanced pancreatic damage.

Helminth Parasites for IBD

Researchers at the University of Iowa College of Medicine are studying the benefits of helminth parasites in treating irritable bowel disease, including ulcerative colitis and Crohn's disease. The intestines house a complex ecosystem of bacteria, viruses and parasites, all of which modulate the intestinal immune system, which is largely governed by Th1 and Th2 cells. Th1 induces inflammation whereas Th2 neutralizes the inflammatory response. Early studies showed a favorable response and an increase in Th2 cells. Clinical trials are currently being conducted to see if additional doses prove beneficial.[9]

Anti–GBM Diseases and Goodpasture Syndrome

Glomerulonephritis mediated by antibodies to the glomerular basement membrane (GBM) is the prototypic human glomerular disease produced by pathogenic antibodies to the intrinsic glomerular components of the kidney. Anti–GBM disease is most often characterized by the abrupt onset of glomerulonephritis with rapidly progressive renal failure.

When anti–GBM disease is associated with pulmonary hemorrhage, this condition is commonly referred to as "Goodpasture's syndrome." The major antigen target of this disease is _3 type IV collagen. The disease may also occur in the transplanted kidneys of patients with Alport's syndrome. Drs. Michael Madaio and Kevin Meyers, at the University of Pennsylvania, are investigating the pathogenesis of this disorder. Their aim is to apply the derived information to better understand the pathogenesis of these diseases and to develop more effective therapies.

FUTURE TREATMENT IMPLICATIONS

Dr. Noel Rose, Professor of Pathology, Molecular Microbiology and Immunology at Johns Hopkins University, emphasizes that virtually all ADs are dependent upon the production of an abnormal population of T lymphocyte cells. "An effective treatment of autoimmune disease," according to Rose, "more efficacious than anything we now have in our armamentarium, would come from finding ways of identifying and turning off these disease-producing T cells."[10]

Identifying and avoiding the environmental triggers of autoimmune disease is one step in modifying these T cells. An awareness of these environmental triggers could offer not only relief from symptoms but hope for permanent remission.

Vaccines as Therapy for MS

In ongoing clinical trials, researchers are using vaccines to stop disease progression in patients with MS. In one trial patients were vaccinated with irradiated autologous myelin basic protein (MBP)-reactive T cells clones. These clones were previously activated in vitro and then irradiated to prevent proliferation. Recipients received a total of three subcutaneous injections of two to four vaccine clones at two and four month intervals. After three vaccinations, there were no MBP-reactive T cells present in the circulation, suggesting a depletion of autoreactive T cells.[11]

Further studies showed clinical improvement over a period of two to three years. Researchers measured several parameters, including exacerbation rate, Expanded Disability Status Scored (EDSS), and quantitative changes in brain lesions as measured by MRI. Compared to control groups in the study, vaccinated patients also experienced fewer relapses.

Vaccinations using T cell receptor (TCR) peptide and, in some cases DNA, are also proving effective in clinical trials with MS patients. TCR peptide vaccines have been proven effective in preventing allergic encephalitis in studies conducted in 1989. DNA vaccines are constructed from DNA encoded the intended antigen. The DNA in the vaccine is taken up by the subject's cells, which then translate and transcribe the DNA information and express the antigen encoded by the injected DNA.[12]

Altered Peptide Ligands

When a T cell receptor encounters a variant of the antigen that it normally recognizes, it induces an aberrant signal within the cell. Regarding autoreactive T cells, which normally produce pro-inflammatory cytokines, the presence of a variant antigen may trigger the production of suppressive cytokines. In one study in which experimental allergic encephalitis was reversed, the altered T cells caused the production of IL-4 instead of interferon-gamma and TNF-alpha. From this study, researchers concluded that paralytic disease induced with a different myelin protein, like proteolysis protein, can be suppressed using an altered peptide legend for myelin basic protein.[13]

Stem Cell Transplantation

The T cell defects responsible for initiating and propagating ADs can, in some instances, be modified through stem cell transplantation combined with high dose chemotherapy. This protocol allows subsequent maturation and outgrowth of transplanted lymphocyte progenitors (early stem cells destined to become T lymphocytes) that would not be capable of reacting against self-antigens.

In one study conducted by the National Institutes of Health, nine SLE patients with severe lupus nephritis, lupus cerebritis, or transverse myelitis unresponsive to conventional therapy were treated with this protocol. Stem cells were harvested from this patient through phlebotomy and later transplanted. The seven patients completing this protocol all achieved remission through a follow-up period of 25 months.[14] In a similar study, researchers from Oxford, U.K., are attempting to restore pancreatic beta cell function in IDDM with stem cell transplants.[15]

Scorpion Venom

Researchers at the University of California–Irvine have recently reported that scorpion venom contains a chemical that suppresses the immune system's T cells. While therapy is not yet available, the researchers estimate that it could prove effective in about 60 different autoimmune disorders.[16] Scorpion stings are painful and have been known to cause death, and AD patients should not seek this treatment unless medical therapy becomes available.

PROMISING THERAPIES

Interferon and monoclonal antibody therapies are currently being developed for use in other autoimmune disorders. For instance, researchers are currently evaluating interferon-alpha-a therapy for Sjögren's syndrome and expect this substance (IF Nalpha) to be available by 2002. In clinical trials, IF Nalpha was shown to increase saliva production without the side effects of pilocarpine.

Monoclonal antibody therapies are currently being developed for IgM neuropathy, celiac disease, RA, Wegener's granulomatosis, polymyositis, MG, pemphigus, AIHA, thrombocytopenia, Graves' disease, thryoiditis, diabetes, amyloidosis, cyroglobulinemia and other disorders.[17]

FINAL THOUGHT

While adding more sand and water may help repair our imaginary sandcastle, protection from the elements is the best defense. Similarly, in dealing with autoimmune disorders, our best defense is an avoidance of environmental triggers, when they can be identified, and strengthening our immune systems through a nutrient rich diet.

11

Resources

Books

The Immune System and Autoimmune Disorders

Dibner, R., and C. Colman, *The Lupus Handbook for Women*, 1994, New York, Simon and Schuster.

Frank, Michael, MD, Editor, *Samter's Immunologic Diseases*, 5th Edition, Vol. 1 and 2, 1995, New York, Little, Brown, and Company.

Lappé, Marc, Ph.D., *The Tao of Immunology: A Revolutionary New Understanding of Our Body's Defenses*, 1997, New York, Plenum Publishing.

Ravicz, Simone, *Thriving with Your Autoimmune Disorder: A Woman's Mind-Body Guide*, 2000, Oakland, CA, New Harbinger Publications, Inc.

Sarno, John E., *The Mindbody Prescription: Healing the Body, Healing the Pain*, 1998, New York, Warner Books.

Environmental Issues

Colborn, Theo, Dumanoski, Dianne, and John Peterson Myers, *Our Stolen Future*, 1997, New York, Plume division of Penguin Publishing.

Fagin, Dan and Marianne Lavelle, and the Center for Public Integrity, *Toxic Deception: How the Chemical Industry Manipulates Science, Bends the Law and Endangers Your Health*, Monroe, Second Edition, 1999, Maine, Common Courage Press.

Krimsky, Sheldon, *Hormonal Chaos: The Scientific and Social Origins of the Environmental Endocrine Hypothesis*, 2000, Baltimore, The Johns Hopkins University Press.

Alternative Resources

Balch, J. F., and P. A. Balch, *Prescription for Nutritional Healing*, Second Edition, 1997, Garden City Park, NY, Avery Publishing Group.

Cousins, Norman, *Head First: The Biology of Hope*, 1989, New York, Dutton Publishing.
Monte, Tom, *The Complete Guide to Natural Healing*, 1997, New York, Perigree Books.
Starck, Marcia, *Handbook of Natural Therapies: Exploring The Spiral of Healing*, 1998, Freedom, CA, The Crossing Press.

Journals and Periodicals

Environmental Health Perspectives and Supplements
National Institute of Environmental Health Sciences
P.O. Box 1233
Research Triangle Park, NC 27709
http://ehis.niehs.nih.gov/

The Lancet

The New England Journal of Medicine
http://www.nejm.org

Science
http://www.sciencemag.org

General Medical Information

Internet Government Resources

Food and Drug Administration
http://www.gda.gov

Government Accounting Office
http://www.gao.gov

Healthfinder
http://www.healthfinder.gov

Medlineplus
http//www.medlineplus.gov

National Library of Medicine
http://www.nlm.nih.gov/nlmhome.html

General Internet Medical Sources

CBS Healthwatch
http://www.healthwatch.medscape.com

The Med Engine!
http://www.themedengine.com

Medscape
This site has a number of divisions
http://www.medscape.com

New England Journal of Medicine
http://www.nejm.org

Reuters Health
http://www.reuthershealth.com

WebMedLit
http://www.webmedlit.com

Organizations and Support Groups

About.com has a number of educational sites and support groups
http://www.about.com

American Autoimmune Related Diseases Association
22100 Gratiot Avenue
East Detroit, Michigan 48021-2227
(810) 776-3900
http://www.aarda.org

Johns Hopkins Vasculitis Center
http://vasculitis.med.jhu.edu/

Mayo University Clinic
http://www.mayo.org/

National Institute of Arthritis and Musculoskeletal and Skin Diseases
National Institute of Health
1 AMS Circle
Bethesda, MD 20892
301-718-6366
http://www.nih.gov/niams

National Institute of Environmental Health Sciences
National Institutes of Health
http://niehs.nih.gov

University of Maryland Autoimmune Disease Center
http://medschool.umaryland.edu/womenshealth/links/auto_immune.html

Specific Autoimmune Disease Organizations

Connective Tissue and Rheumatological Disorders

American College of Rheumatology
60 Executive Park South, Suite 150
Atlanta, GA 30329
(404) 633-3777

Arthritis Foundation
1650 Bluegrass Lakes Pkwy.
Alpharetta, GA 30009
(800) 283-7800
http://www.arthritis.org

Lupus Foundation of America
1300 Piccard Drive, Suite 100
Rockville, MD 20850-4303
(800) 558-0121
http://www.lupus.org/lupus

Lupus Living Support Group
http://www.medakate.org/lupus.html

National Institute of Arthritis and Musculoskeletal and Skin Diseases
   (NIAMS)
1 AMS Circle
Bethesda, MD 20892-3675
http://www.nih.gov/niams/healthinfo/

National Sjögren's Syndrome Association
5815 N. Black Canyon Highway, Suite 103
Phoenix, AZ 85015-2200
(602) 433-9844
http://www.sjogrens.org

Sjögren's Syndrome Foundation
333 N. Broadway
Jericho, NY 11753
1-800-4-SJOGRENS OR (516) 933-6365
http://www.sjogrens.com

Sjögren's Syndrome Guide for Patients: Scripps Clinic
LaJolla, California
http://www.dry.org

The S.L.E. Foundation
149 Madison Avenue, Suite 205
New York, NY 10016
(800) 754-8787
http://www.lupus.org/lupus

Spondylitis Association of America
P.O. Box 5872
Sherman Oaks, CA 91413
(800) 777-8189 or (888) 777-1594
http://www.spondylitis.org

United Scleroderma Foundation
89 Newbury Street, Suite 201
Danvers, MA 01923
(800) 722-HOPE
Fax: (978) 750-9902
http://www.scleroderma.org

Gastrointestinal and Liver Disorders

American Liver Foundation
1425 Pompton Avenue
Cedar Grove, NJ 07009
800-465-4837
http://sadieo.ucsf.edu/ALF/alffinal/homepagealf.html

Crohn's and Colitis Foundation of America
386 Park Avenue South, 17th Floor
New York, NY 10016-8804
(800) 343-3637
http://www.ccfa.org

Neurological and Neuromuscular Disorders

Guillian-Barré Syndrome Foundation International
P. O. Box 262
Wynnewood, PA 19096
(610) 667-0131
http://www.gbs.org

Myasthenia Gravis Foundation of America
222 S. Riverside Plaza, Suite 1540
Chicago, IL 60606
(800) 541-5454
http://www.med.unc.edu/mgfa

Myositis Association of America
1420 Huron Court
Harrisonburg, VA 22801
(540) 433-7686
http://www.myositis.org

National Institute of Arthritis and Musculoskeletal and Skin Diseases
   (NIAMS)
http://www.nih.gov/niams

National Institute of Neurological Disorders and Stroke
Office of Scientific and Health Reports
P. O. Box 5801
Bethesda, MD 20824
(301) 496-5751
http://www.ninds.nih.gov/hlthinhp.htm

National Multiple Sclerosis Society
733 Third Avenue, 6th Floor
New York, NY 10017-3288
(800) 344-4867
http://www.nmss.org

Dermatological and Pemphigoid Disorders

The Johns Hopkins Pemphigus Research Center
1620 McElderry Street
Baltimore, MD 21205
410-955-3644
http://www.med.jhu.edu/pemphigus/

National Alopecia Areata Foundation
710 C Street, Suite 11
San Rafael, CA 94901-3853
(415) 456-4644

The National Pemphigus Foundation
Atrium Plaza, Suite 203
828 San Pablo Avenue
Albany, CA 94707

510-527-4970
http://www.pemphigus.org/foundation.htm

National Psoriasis Foundation
66000 SW 92nd Avenue, Suite 300
Portland, OR 97223
(800) 723-9166
http://www.psoriasis.org

National Vitiligo Foundation
P.O. Box 6337
Tyler, TX 75703
(903) 531-0074
http://www.nvfi.org

Digestive, Diabetes and Kidney Disorders

Juvenile Diabetes Foundation International
120 Wall Street
New York, NY 10005-4001
(800) JDF-CURE or (800) 533-2873

National Institutes of Health's National Institute of Diabetes, Digestive and
    Kidney Diseases (NIDDK)
Information Clearinghouse
1 Information Way
Bethesda, MD 20892-3560
http://www.niddk.nih.gov/

Wegener's Foundation
3705 South George Mason Drive, Suite 1813
Falls Church, VA 22041
(703) 931-5852

Wegener's Granulomatosis Support Group
P.O. Box 28660
Kansas City, MO 64188-8668
(800) 277-9474
http://www.wgsg.org

Autoimmune Endocrine Disorders

American Association of Clinical Endocrinologists
1000 Riverside Avenue, Suite 205

Jacksonville, FL 32204
Phone: (904) 353-7878
http://www.aace.com

American Diabetes Association
1660 Duke Street
Alexandria, VA 22314
(800) 232-3472
http://www.diabetes.org

American Foundation of Thyroid Patients
P.O. Box 820195
Houston, TX 77282-0195
Phone: (281) 496-4460 or 1-888-996-4460
Email: *thyroid@flash.net*
http://www.thyroidfoundation.org

American Thyroid Association
Montefiore Medical Center
111 East 210th Street, Room 311
Bronx, NY 10467
Phone: (718) 882-6047
Fax: (718) 882-6085
http://www.thyroid.org

Broda Barnes Foundation for Thyroid Disorders
P. O. Box 98
Trumbell, CT 06611
(203) 261-2101
http://www.brodabarnes.org

Endocrine Society
4350 East West Highway, Suite 500
Bethesda, MD 20814-4410
Phone: (301) 941-0200
http://www.endo-society.org/index.htm

Gland Central for Thyroid Disorders
http://www.glandcentral.com

Hypoparathyroidism Organization
2835 Salmon
Idaho Falls, ID 83406
(208) 524-3857
http://www.hypoparathyroidism.org

National Graves' Disease Foundation
P.O. Box 1969
Brevard, NC 28712
(828) 877-5251
http://www.ngdf.org

The Thyroid Foundation of America
40 Parkman Street
Boston, MA 02114-2698
(800) 832-8321
http://www.tsh.org

Thyroid Society for Education and Research
7515 South Main Street, Suite 545
Houston, TX 77030
http://www.the-thyroid-society.org

Rare Diseases

Behçet's Association
PO Box 54063
Minneapolis, MN
(800) BEHCETS
http://www.w2.com/behcets.html

Behçets Organization Worldwide
www.alexknight.clara.net/Behcets-syndrome/

National Organization for Rare Disorders
P. O. Box 8923
New Fairfield, CT 06812-1783
(800) 999-6673
http://www.nord-rdb.com/~orphan

Office of Rare Diseases, National Institutes of Health
Bldg. 31 Rm. 1B03
31 Center Drive
Bethesda, MD 20892
(301) 402-4336
http://cancernet.nci.nih.gov/ord/p_home.htm

Peyronie's Disease
http://www.urologychannel.com/peyronies/index.shtml/
http://www.malehealthcenter.com/peyron.htm

Internet Sites with Laboratory Test Information

http://216.117.138.253/lab/cwpl.html

http://hsc.virginia.edu/medicine/clinical/pathology/labtests/index.htm

http://www.ariess.com/s-crina/tests-bloodindex.htm

http://www.cap.org

http://www.cat.cc.md.us/~gkaiser/lecguide/unit3/u3iibc.html

http://www.neosoft.com/~uthman/lab_test.html

http://www.njc.org

http://www.pathguy.com/erf/lectures/profilin.htm

Laboratory Tests and Pharmaceutical Information

http://www.pharma-lexicon.com

Environmental Resources ·

Feat Daily Newsletter
Sacramento, California
http://www.feat.org

The National Coalition Against the Misuse of Pesticides
701 E. Street SE, Suite 200
Washington, DC 20003
202-543-5450

National Vaccine Information Center
221 Lawyers Road
Vienna, VA 22180
800 909-SHOT
http://www.909shot.com

The Pesticide Education Center
P.O. Box 420870
San Francisco, CA 94142
415-391-8511

Rachel Carson Council
8940 Jones Mill Road
Chevy Chase, MD 20815
301-652-1877

Clinical Trial Information

Center Watch
Clinical Trials Listing Service
http://centerwatch.com/studies

Clinical Studies
http://www.clinicaltrials.com
http://www.veritasmedicine.com/index.cfm

Government Associated Trials
http://www.clinicaltrials.gov
http://www.nimh.nih.gov/studies/index.cfm

Infertility Associated with Autoimmune Diseases

Finch University
http://www.repro-med.net/papers/thyroid.html

Information on Prescription Drugs

http://www.medbroadcast.com

http://www.shoppersdrugmart.ca

Low Cost Prescription Programs

http://www.NeedyMeds.com

http://www.sunflower.org/~cfsdays/freedrug.htm

http://www.themedicineprogram.com

Alternative Medicine Resources

Acupuncture.com
http://www.acupuncture.com

American Association of Naturopathic Physicians
2366 Eastlake Avenue East, Suite 322
Seattle, WA 98102
(206) 323-7610
http://www.naturopathic.org/

Health Coach
http://www.bcn.net/~stoll/

The Life Extension Foundation
http://www.lef.org

Nutrition and Allergies

Food Allergy Network
10400 Eaton Place #107
Fairfax, VA 22030-2208
(800) 929-4040
http://www.foodallergy.org

Rheumatoid Arthritis Nutrition
http://www.healingwithnutrition.com/disease/arthritis

Road Back Foundation Patient Information Center
http://www.roadback.org

National Institute of Health Office of Dietary Supplements
http://dietary-supplements.info.nigh.gov/

National Women's Health Information Center
Office of Women's Health
U.S. Department of Health and Human Services
(800) 994-WOMAN
http://www.4women.gov/

Touch Therapy

Health Touch Therapy
http://www.healthtouch.com

Herbal Therapy

American Botanical Council Online
http://www.herbalgram.org/

Herb Research Foundation
1007 Pear Street, Suite 200
Boulder, CO 80302
(800) 748-2617
http://www.herbs.org

Amalgam Filling Information

Environmental Dental Association
9974 Scripps Ranch Blvd. Suite 36
San Diego, CA 92131
(800) 388-8124

Huggins Diagnostic Center
5080 List Dr.
Colorado Springs, CO 80919
(719) 548-1600

Glossary

Adaptive immunity   Also known as acquired immunity; immune response initiated by a specific stimulus that T cells have been programmed to respond to

Addison's disease   Autoimmune condition of adrenal gland insufficiency

Adenoma   Tissue growth or nodule derived from glandular tissue or from recognizable glandular structures

Adrenal glands   Endocrine glands located on top of the kidneys that secrete several important hormones including cortisol into the blood circulation

AIH   *see* Autoimmune hepatitis

AIHA   *see* Autoimmune hemolytic anemia

AITD   *see* Autoimmune thyroid disease

Allele   One of a pair of genes normally occupying a certain gene locus; homozygous alleles refer to identical alleles sharing a locus, whereas heterozygous alleles refer to different alleles occupying a locus

Allergic rhinitis   Inflammation of the mucous membrane of the nose caused by a hypersensitivity reaction to environmental substances such as pollen or mold

Alloantibodies   Antibodies produced in response to exposure of foreign antigens of the same species, such as antibodies directed against other blood type antigens such as Rh or Kell.

Alopecia areata   Autoimmune disorder characterized by baldness, including loss of axillary hair.

Amenorrhea   Absence of menstrual periods

ANA   *see* Antinuclear antibodies

Anaphylaxis   An immediate hypersensitivity reaction characterized by local reactions, such as urticaria (hives) and angiodema (redness and swelling) or systemic reactions in the respiratory tract, cardiovascular system, gastrointestinal tract and skin.

Antibody   Specific immunoglobulin produced by B lymphocytes in response to an antigenic challenge; antibodies can be found in blood and other body fluids and milk; antibodies are capable of binding and neutralizing the antigens that stimulated their production

Antigenic   Substance capable of acting as an antigen and eliciting an immune system response

Antineutrophil cytoplasmic antibodies (ANCA)   Autoantibodies against the neutrophilic cytoplasm of white blood cells having several subtypes, including P-ANCA and C-ANCA; seen in vasculitis, Wegener's granulomatosus, and other autoimmune disorders

Antinuclear antibodies (ANA)   Autoantibody directed against the cell nucleus of various tissue organ; while ANA are commonly associated with systemic lupus, they may be found in many other autoimmune disorders, and in low titers, they're seen in some normal individuals; ANA are further differentiated by the type of staining pattern they demonstrate in testing

Antiphospholipid syndrome (APS)   Autoimmune condition associated with the presence of antiphosphopholipid antibodies (anticardiolipin antibodies and lupus anticoagulant) responsible for deep vein thrombosis, strokes and miscarriages

Antithyroid drugs   Medications such as propylthiouracil (PTU) or methimazole that interfere with iodine absorption by thyroid cells, which ultimately diminishes the amount of thyroid hormone produced by the thyroid gland

Apoptosis   Normal condition of programmed cell death

Arthralgia   Pain related to joint inflammation

Articular   Referring to the joints of the body

Ataxia   Irregularity of muscular action or faulty muscular coordination

ATD   *see* Antithyroid drugs

Atherosclerosis   Condition marked by loss of elasticity or hardening of the walls of the blood vessels

Atopic eczema   Inflammation of the epidermal layer of the skin characterized by redness, itching, and weeping resulting from a hypersensitivity reaction

Atrophy   Wasting or lack of cellular growth seen in tissues and organs

Autoantibodies   Antibodies directed against the body's own tissues, cells and protein molecules; see chapter 6 for an extensive list of autoantibodies and the diseases they're associated with

Autoimmune disease (AD)   Disorder caused by an immune system defect that causes the immune system to attack self molecules

Autoimmune hemolytic anemia (AIHA)   Autoimmune condition of red blood cell destruction

Autoimmune hepatitis (AIH)   Condition with two subtypes in which hepatocytes (liver cells) are destroyed by an autoimmune process

Autoimmune thyroid disease   One of a number of different autoimmune conditions affecting the thyroid causing symptoms of hypothyroidism, hyperthyroidism, and thyroid failure

Autoimmunity   Condition in which an individual has positive autoantibody titers but no symptoms of disease

Autoreative cells   Intermediate step in autoantibody production; autoreactive cells target self components; autoreactive cells either become destroyed by other cells or go on to form autoantibodies

B lymphocyte cells   Type of immune system cell involved in antibody production

Bilateral   Affecting both sides of the body equally

Biliary   Pertaining to bile, bile ducts or the gallbladder

Bilirubin   Breakdown product of erythrocyte (red blood cell) catabolism; high levels are deposited in lipid-rich tissues, such as the eyes and skin, causing jaundice or icterus, and in the brain disrupting normal brain function

Binding proteins   Proteins normally found in the blood that bind substances such as hormones, transporting and carrying these substances to cell receptors located throughout the body

Bone marrow   Structure within bone that contains blood forming tissues

C3   The most abundant and important component of complement

C-Reactive protein (CRP)   A nonspecific protein that rises in response to inflammation

Campylobacter jejuni   Bacterial pathogen that is the most commonly reported cause of foodborne infection in the United States

Cardiolipin   Phospholipid occurring primarily in the inner membrane of mitochondrial cells

CAT or CT   Computed axial tomography, an imaging technique

Catecholamines   Biologically active amine compounds, including epinephrine and norepinephrine, that influence the nervous and cardiovascular systems, metabolic rate and temperature, and smooth muscle contractions

Cell   Basic building block of living organisms

Cell-mediated immunity   Immunity initiated by T cells and macrophages

Centromere   The constricted portion of a chromosome

Cerebrospinal fluid (CSF)   Clear fluid formed by the choroids plexus in the ventricles of the brain and found within the subarachnoid space, the central canal of the spinal cord and the four ventricles of the brain

Cholestasis   Blockage or suppression of bile flow

Chromosome   Found in the cell nucleus, chromosomes contain specific regions of DNA; the human body has 23 pairs of chromosomes that together contain the body's genetic code

CIDP   Chronic inflammatory demyelinating polyneuropathy

Cirrhosis   Chronic liver disease in which fibrous tissue invades and replaces normal tissue

Collagen   Protein found in skin, tendons, bone, and cartilage

Collagen disease   Connective tissue disorder

Complement   Group of proteins present in the blood that can produce inflammations and cell lysis when activated; some bacteria activate complement directly while others do so with the help of antibody; complement works in a cascading sequence of complement subtypes

Coombs test *see* Direct antiglobulin test

Corticosteroid   Steroid hormones produced by the adrenal glands

Costochondritis   Condition of musculoskeletal pain and tenderness of the chest wall, without swelling, caused by inflammation of the rib cartilage and small muscles between the ribs, often associated with rheumatic autoimmune diseases, especially lupus; lupus chest pain

Cross-reactivity   A condition in which some of the determinants of an antigen are shared by similar antigenic determinants on the surface of apparently unrelated molecules and a proportion of these antigens interact with the antigen that they mimic

Cryoglobulin   Abnormal protein that precipitates at cold temperatures but redissolves at warm temperatures

CSF *see* Cerebrospinal fluid

Cytokine   Immune system messenger chemical that regulates the intensity and duration of immune responses; includes interferons, interleukins and various growth factors; also known as lymphokines and chemokines

Cytomegalovirus (CMV)   Type of herpes virus that can cause congenital infections in the newborn and a clinical syndrome resembling infectious mononucleosis

Cytotoxic   Capable of causing cellular damage or destruction

Cytotoxic T lymphocytes (CTLs)   Immune system cells capable of destroying other cells

Dendrites   Weakly phagocytic cells found in the epidermis and non-phagocytic cells found in the lymphoid follicles of the spleen and lymph nodes. These cells may be the main agent of T cell stimulation

Dendritic   Threadlike extensions of the cytoplasm of neurons

Deoxyribonucleic acid (DNA)   Nucleic acid that forms the main structure of genes

Dermatitis herpetiformis   Autoimmune disorder characterized by gluten sensitivity and a chronic skin disorder, including eruptions, blistering and discoloration; Durhing's disease

Dermatomyositis   Inflammatory collagen disease in which the skin, subcutaneous tissues, and muscles are involved; may progress to muscle necrosis

Diethylstilbesterol (DES)   Synthetic, non-steroidal estrogen compound with estrogenic activity greater than estrone

Diplopia   Double vision

Direct antiglobulin test (DAT)   Blood test used to determine the presence of autoantibodies or complement coating red blood cells

Discoid lupus   Benign dermatological condition characterized by the lupus rash, but without systemic disease development

Drug related lupus (DRL)   Lupus disorder similar to that of systemic lupus, although joint pain and kidney involvement are rarely seen, caused in reaction to a medication; condition resolves when drug is discontinued

Dysphagia   Difficulty swallowing

Dyspnea   Shortness of breath

Dystonia   Uncontrolled erratic movement related to disordered muscle tonicity

ECHO   Echoenceophalogram scan.

Ectopic   Cells or tissue developing away from their customary location

Edema   Accumulation of fluid in tissues causing swelling

EEG   Electroencephalogram

EMG   Electromyography

Endocarditis   Inflammation of the inner lining of the heart (endocardium)

Endocrine   Referring to the endocrine system of glands that release hormones directly into the circulation

Endogenous   Developing or originating within the organism or arising from causes within the organism

ENG   Electronystagmography

Enteropathy   Intestinal disorder, such as gluten sensitivity enteropathy

Environmental   Factors originating outside of the body, such as those attributed to the elements and nature and also synthetic chemicals, foods, infectious agents and emotions

Epidemiology   Study of infectious diseases or conditions in many individuals in the same geographic location at the same time

Epithelial cells   Type of cell forming the lining of internal and external tissue surfaces or composing a body structure such as glandular epithelium

Erythematosus   Characterized by erythema or redness of the skin

Erythrocyte   Red blood cell

Estrogen   Pertaining collectively to the six different female sex hormone derivatives having estrogenic properties, the most common being estriol, estradiol and estrone.

Etiology   Pertaining to the causes of disease

Exophthalmos   Protrusion of the eyeball from the orbit; proptosis

Extracellular   Outside of the blood cells and in the peripheral circulation

Extravascular hemolysis   Phagocytizing and catabolizing of erythrocytes by the mononuclear-phagocytic cells of the immune system, causing cell rupture or lysis

Febrile   Pertaining to an elevation of body temperature; fever

Fibroblast   Immature fiber-producing cell of connective tissue capable of differentiating into a cartilage-forming cell, a collagen-forming cell, or a bone-forming cell (osteoblast)

Fibromyalgia   Condition characterized by muscle and joint pain, including myofascial pain, which is thought to have an autoimmune component

GBM   Glomerular basement membrane

GBS   *see* Guillain-Barré syndrome

GD   *see* Graves' disease

Gene   Short pieces of DNA which contain coded instructions

Genetic susceptibility   Having a certain combination of genes that increases the likelihood of developing certain diseases

Glomerulonephritis   Autoimmune kidney disorder associated with inflammation of the small convoluted mass of capillaries necessary for blood circulation in the kidneys.

Glomerulus   One of the blood filtering structures which comprise the nephron, the functional unit in the kidney

GO   *see* Graves' ophthalmopathy

Graves' disease (GD)   Autoimmune hyperthyroid condition that may also affect the eyes, skin and muscular system

Graves' ophthalmopathy (GO)   Eye disorder associated with Graves' disease which has two subtypes, a spastic condition caused by excess thyroid hormone and a congestive infiltrative disorder caused by immune system changes; typical symptoms include diplopia, exophthalmos, dry eyes and optic nerve compression

Guillain-Barré syndrome   Autoimmune disorder affecting the nervous system; also called acute idiopathic polyneuritis

Haplotype   Genes occurring together that may be inherited together as pairs

Hapten   Antigenic determinant of low molecular weight that can act as an immunogen when coupled to an immogenic carrier molecule; drugs can act as haptens and bind to the surface of red blood cells, altering their immune properties

Hashimoto's thyroiditis   Autoimmune hypothyroid disease responsible for most instances of hypothyroidism in the United States

Hashitoxicosis   Condition in which patients with Hashimoto's thyroiditis have simultaneous periods of hyperthyroidism

Heliotrope rash   Purplish swelling in orbital area seen in dermatomyositis

HLA antigens   Genetic markers of the major histocompatibility complex in man expressed on the body's white blood cells

Hormone   Chemical substance secreted by glands that affects the functions of specifically receptive organs or tissues

HT   *see* Hashimoto's thyroiditis

Humoral   Pertaining to any fluid substance normally found in the body

Humoral immunity   Form of defense represented by antibodies and other soluble, extracellular factors in the blood and lymphatic fluid

Hypercalcemia   Excess level of ionized calcium in the blood

Hyperplasia   Abnormal cell multiplication; erratic cellular growth

Hypertrophy   Abnormal increase in cell size

Hypocalcemia   Decreased level of ionized calcium in the blood

IDDM   *see* Insulin dependent diabetes mellitus

IFN   *see* Interferon

IL   *see* Interleukin

Immune complex   Combination of a linked antigen with its specific antibody; immune complexes can be small and soluble or large and precipitating

Immune system   Group of organs and cells that work together to protect the body from foreign substances and infected and malignant cell growth

Immunity   Condition of being resistant, conferred by acquired or passive antibody production

Immunoglobulin (Ig)   Protein from which antibodies are derived; used synonymously for all globulins having antibody activity; there are 5 classes of immunoglobulins with IgG being the most abundant

Immunosuppressant   Drug, chemical or other mechanism that prevents the immune system from recognizing and responding to foreign antigens

Immunosuppression   Repression of the normal adaptive immune response through the use of drugs, chemicals or other means

Insulin dependent diabetes mellitus (IDDM)   Disorder of erratic blood sugar levels due to impaired insulin production caused by autoantibodies that destroy the insulin-producing islet cells of the pancreas; type 1 or juvenile diabetes

Interferon (IFN)   Cytokine with many functions including defense against viruses

Interleukin   Cytokine with diverse immunologic and inflammatory functions

Islet of Langerhans   Any of the clusters of endocrine cells in the pancreas that are specialized to secrete insulin, somatostatin, or glucagon

ITP   Idiopathic thrombocytopenic purpura; autoimmune platelet deficiency

Leukocyte   White blood cell found in the normal circulation that functions as part of the immune system in antigen recognition and antibody formation

Leukocytosis   Marked increase in total circulating white blood cells

Leukopenia   Marked decrease in total circulating white blood cells

Lumbar Puncture (LP)   Procedure in which cerebrospinal fluid is withdrawn from the spinal cord in the lumbar or lower back region

Lupus   Referring to the characteristic rash seen in patients with lupus disorders, which was considered wolf-like when first identified; referring to any of the lupus disorders, such as discoid lupus, systemic lupus erythematosus and neonatal transient lupus

Lymph node   Accumulation of lymphoid tissue organized as definite lymphoid organs situated along the course of the lymphatic vessels

Lymphatics   System of lymphatic vessels that carry lymph fluid through the body

Lymphocyte   Small leukocyte found in lymph nodes and the circulating blood with two major subtypes known as T and B cells

Lymphoma   Solid, malignant tumor of the lymph nodes and associated tissues of the bone marrow

Macrophage   Large mononuclear phagocytic cell of the tissues that exists as either a wandering type or a fixed type that lines the capillaries and sinuses of organs such as the bone marrow, spleen, and lymph nodes; macrophages phagocytize, process and present antigens to T cells and they engulf, thereby removing, damaged and infected tissue cells

Major histocompatibility complex (MHC)   Immune system genes located on the short arm of chromosome 6 that regulate the immune response

Mesangial proliferative glomerulonephritis   Inflammation of the kidney glomerulus due to abnormal IgM antibody deposits in the mesangial layer of the glomerular capillary

MG *see* Myasthenia gravis

MHC *see* Major histocompatibility complex

Mitral valve   Valve between the heart's left atrium and left ventricle that prevents blood from flowing back into the atrium when the ventricle contracts

Molecular mimicry   Cross-reactivity between an antigen and a tissue component

Monoclonal antibody   Purified immunoglobulins produced by cells that are cloned from a single fusion-type hybridoma cell; monoclonal antibodies are directed exclusively against antigens derived from a single cell line

Monocyte   Type of leukocyte found in the peripheral blood with phagocytic properties

MRI   Magnetic resonance imaging

Multiple sclerosis (MS)   Autoimmune disease characterized by deterioration of the myelin sheath covering nerves, resulting in impaired nerve transmission

Myasthenia gravis (MG)   Autoimmune disease of impaired transmission of motor nerve impulses, characterized by episodic weakness and muscle fatigue

Myelin   Substance making up the protective sheath of nerve axons.

Myxedema   Condition of hypothyroidism characterized by thickening of the skin, blunting of the senses and intellect, and labored speech

Natural killer (NK) cells   Population of effector lymphocytes that produce cytokines and cause cell destruction

Necrosis   The death of cells or a localized group of cells or tissue

Nephritis   Inflammation of the nephrons, the primary functional units of the kidney

Nephrotic syndrome   Disorder of the kidneys characterized by a decreased concentration of albumin in the circulating blood, marked edema, increased protein in the urine (proteinuria) and increased susceptibility to infection

Neuropathy   Nerve inflammation

Neutropenia   Marked decrease in neutrophils (granulocytic leukocytes)

NIEHS   National Institute of Environmental Health Sciences

NIH   National Institutes of Health

Oncovirus   Retrovirus of the subfamily *Oncovirinae*, capable of altering its messenger RNA and producing tumors

Parotid gland   Largest of the three salivary glands, located near the ear

Paroxysmal cold hemoglobinuria (PCH)   Condition of red blood cell destruction caused by an IgG protein that reacts with the erythrocytes in colder parts of the body and subsequently causes complement components to irreversibly bind to erythrocytes; commonly seen as an acute transient condition occurring secondary to a viral infection

PBC Primary biliary cirrhosis

Pericarditis Inflammation of the serous membrane lining the sac surrounding the heart (pericardium) and the origins of the great vessels; pericardial swelling in pericarditis can mimic a heart attack, appearing in the middle or left front of the chest, possibly radiating back the shoulder, and affected by changes in position; left untreated, pericarditis can cause scar tissue to form in the pericardial sac which can eventually cause restriction of the heart itself

PETT Positron Emission Transaxial Tomography

Phagocytes Immune system cells capable of ingesting and destroying particles, including microbes and infected cells; macrophages are phagocytes

Platelet *see* Thrombocyte

Pleuritis Inflammation and swelling of the pleura, the serosal membrane surrounding the lungs; pleurisy; the amount of pleural fluid in pleuritis may increase as the membrane swells

Phagocyte Any cell capable of engulfing and destroying foreign particles such as bacteria or other infected or damaged cells

Plasma Straw colored fluid component of blood in circulating or anticoagulated blood specimens

PM Polymyositis

PNI Psychoneuroimmunology; the study of the relationship between the nervous, immune and endocrine systems

Polyarteritis nodosa Inflammatory process affecting the layers of small and medium sized arteries; manifested by various symptoms including febrile reactions

Polyendocrinopathies Autoimmune disorder involving several different endocrine glands; polyglandular syndromes

Primary lymphoid tissue Bone marrow or thymus, the sites of lymphocyte origin and maturation

Prognosis Forecast of the probable outcome of a condition or disease

Progressive systemic sclerosis (PSS) Autoimmune disorder characterized by loss of tissue elasticity throughout the body that advances in severity over time

PSC Primary sclerosing cholangitis

Psychoneuroimmunology (PNI) Study of the relationship between the central nervous system, the endocrine system and the immune system; the mind-body connection

Psychosomatic Of or pertaining to a physical disorder that is caused or notably influenced by emotional factors

Purpura Extensive area of red or purple skin discolorations

RA *see* Rheumatoid arthritis

Raynaud's phenomenon Condition of episodic constriction of small arteries of the extremities (usually fingers and toes) induced by cold temperatures or emotional stress that would not affect an unafflicted person; symptoms include a pale appearance (blanching) and numbness followed by redness and tingling or a swollen, red, painful condition; primary Raynaud's phenomenon

Raynaud's syndrome   More serious, less common form of Raynaud's phenomenon that usually accompanies another autoimmune conditions, such as scleroderma, rheumatoid arthritis or systemic lupus; occurs more often in males, pre-pubertal girls and women older than 35; secondary Raynaud's phenomenon

Retrovirus   RNA virus that uses reverse transcriptase enzyme for its replication

Rheumatoid arthritis (RA)   Autoimmune connective tissue disorder associated with the presence of autoantibodies to IgG (rheumatoid factor or RF) causing symmetrical joint pain.

Rheumatoid factor   Immunoglobulin, usually IgM, directed against IgG, often seen in patients with rheumatoid arthritis and other connective tissue disorders

Ribonucleic Acid (RNA)   Messenger protein used in the intermediate steps leading to DNA production

Riedel's thyroiditis   Rare, chronic proliferating inflammatory disorder usually affecting one thyroid lobe, although it may extend to both lobes and also the trachea

Serositis   Inflammation of the membrane consisting of mesothelium, a thin layer of connective tissue, having lines enclosing the body cavities

Sjögren's syndrome (SS)   Autoimmune disorder manifested by ocular and oral dryness and enlargement of the parotid glands; systemic form includes the glands of the vagina and stomach mucosa and chronic polyarthritis

SLE   *see* Systemic lupus erythematosus

Spleen   Large organ located in the upper left quadrant of abdomen under the ribs; functions to filter blood and store mononuclear-phagocytic cells

Splenomegaly   Condition of having an enlarged spleen

Subclinical   Mild disease form usually without symptoms but characterized by abnormal laboratory tests

Synovitis   Inflammation of a synovial membrane; this condition is usually painful, particularly during motion

Synovium   Interior area of joints containing synovial fluid

Systemic lupus erythematosus (SLE)   Autoimmune disorder that can affect practically every organ in the body marked by cellular destruction and immune complex deposits

T lymphocyte cell   Type of white blood cell responsible for the cellular immune response and involved in the regulation of antibody production

Telangiectasia   Permanent dilation of preexisting blood vessels, creating small focal red lesions

Thrombocyte   Blood component distinct from blood cells derived from the megakaryocyte system essential for proper blood clotting; platelets

Thrombocytopenia   Severe deficiency of circulating blood thrombocytes

Thymoma   Tumor derived from the epithelial or lymphoid elements of the thymus

Thymosin   Humoral factor secreted by the thymus which promotes the growth of peripheral lymphoid tissue

Thymus   Primary lymphoid tissue located beneath the sternum (breastbone) responsible for the maturation and storage of T lymphocytes

Thyroid hormone   Hormone produced in the body by the binding of the mineral iodine with the amino acid tyrosine; the two most predominant thyroid hormones include tetraiodothyronine (thyroxine, T4) and tri-iodothyronine (T3)

Thyroid stimulating hormone (TSH)   Hormone released by the pituitary gland that regulates thyroid hormone levels in the blood

Titer   Concentration or strength of an antibody expresses as the highest dilution of serum that causes reactivity, e.g., 1:4, 1:8, etc.

Transcription   Synthesis of RNA from a DNA template

Trypanasoma cruzi   Organism responsible for the development of Chagas' disease

TSH receptor antibodies   Thyroid autoantibodies that target TSH receptor protein; there are three subtypes, stimulating TSH receptor antibodies that cause hyperthyroidism in patients with Graves' disease, blocking antibodies that prevent TSH from acting with the cell receptor, causing autoimmune hypothyroidism, and binding antibodies which may either stimulate the cell receptor or bind with the receptor without causing effects

Ultrasonography (ultrasound)   Diagnostic imaging technique utilizing reflected ultrasonic waves to delineate, measure, or examine internal body structures or organs

Urticaria   Hives

Vaccine   Suspension of killed or attenuated (inactivated) infectious agents administered for the purpose of establishing resistance to a particular disease by inducing antibody production

Vasculitis   Inflammation of blood vessels, impairing normal circulation

Vitiligo   Autoimmune disorder characterized by patches of unpigmented skin

Yin and Yang   Opposing polarities such as hot and cold that govern man as well as the universe; from Eastern medicine

Xenobiotics   Non-living substances capable of causing biologic effects

Notes

Chapter 1

1. Schoen, Frederick, MD, PhD, Managing Editor, *Robbins Pathologic Basis of Disease*, Fifth Edition, Philadelphia, W. B. Saunders, 1994, 197.
2. Pimentel, David, PhD, et al., "Ecology of Increasing Disease: Population Growth and Environmental Degradation," in *BioScience*, Oct. 1998.
3. Yazbak, F. Edward, MD, FAAP, "Autism 99: A National Emergency" via the Internet, www.garynull.com/Documents/autism_99.htm
4. Wakefield, AJ, SH Murch, et al., "Ileal-lymphoid-nodular hyperplasia, non-specific colitis, and pervasive developmental disorder in children," *Lancet*. 1998 Feb. 28;351(9103): 637–42.
5. Tucker, Miriam, "MMR Vaccine on Trial at Congressional Hearing" in *Pediatric News* 34(5):8, 2000 International Medical News Group via Medscape, the Internet.
6. "NIEHS Investigates Link Between Children, the Environment and Neurotoxicity," *Environmental Health Perspectives*, Environews, June, 2001, Volume 109(6): A257–A258.
7. Segni, M., et al., "Specialized Features of Graves' Disease in Early Childhood," Department of Pediatrics, University La Sapienza, Rome, Italy, *Thyroid*, September, 1999;9(9):871–877.

Chapter 2

1. Lappé, Marc, PhD, *The Tao of Immunology, A Revolutionary New Understanding of Our Body's Defenses*, New York, Plenum, 1997, 113.
2. *Ibid.*, 48.
3. "Understanding Autoimmune Disease," publication of the National Institute of Health via the Internet, http://www.niad.nih.gov/publications/autoimmune/autoimmune. htm, Dec 1998, 3.

Chapter 3

1. Ojeda, Sergio, "Organization of the Endocrine System," *Textbook of Endocrine Physiology*, 3.
2. Moore, Elaine A., *Graves' Disease, A Practical Guide*, Jefferson, NC, McFarland & Company, 2001.
3. Op. cit., Ojeda, 4.

4. *Ibid.*

5. Locke, Steven and Douglas Colligan, *The Healer Within: The New Medicine of Mind and Body,* New York, Dutton, 38.

6. Op. cit., Lappé, 55.

7. Fox, Maggie, "Study May Force Re-Think on Rheumatoid Arthritis," *Reuters Health,* Washington, August 1, 2000.

8. Warren, Jeffrey, "Cytokines in Autoimmune Disease," *Clinics In Laboratory Medicine, Progress and Controversies in Autoimmune Disease Testing,* Philadelphia, W. B. Saunders, Sept., 1997, 547–558.

9. Centofani, Marjorie, "Salmonella's Molecular Mimics May Spark Arthritis, Study Shows," *The Gazette Online,* John Hopkins University, February 7, 2000, Vol. 29 (21), 1.

10. Op. cit., Lappé, 104.

11. Reines, Philip, "Hypothesis Bystanders or Bad Seeds? Many Autoimmune Target Cells May Be Transforming to Cancer and Signaling 'Danger' to the Immune System," *Autoimmunity,* 2001, 33(2): 121–134.

Chapter 4

1. Greenspan, Frances, *Basic and Clinical Endocrinology,* 3rd Ed., Appleton & Laange, Norwalk, CT, 1991, 221.

2. Whitacre, Caroline C., Stephen C. Reingold, Patricia O'Looney, et al., The Task Force on Gender, Multiple Sclerosis and Autoimmunity, "A Gender Gap in Autoimmunity, Sex Differences in Autoimmune Disease: Focus on Multiple Sclerosis" in *Science Magazine,* February, 1999, 1–24 via the internet, http://www.sciencemag.org/feature/data/983519.shl.

Chapter 5

1. "Understanding Autoimmune Disease," National Institutes of Health, December 1998, 10; via the internet, http://www.niaid.nih.gov/publications/autoimmune/auto immune.htm.

2. "EPA's Problems with Collection and Management of Scientific Data and Its Efforts to Address Them," *General Accounting Office Report,* 12 May 1995, 4.

3. Ravicz, Simone, *Thriving with Your Autoimmune Disorder, A Woman's Mind-Body Guide,* Oakland, CA, New Harbinger Publications, 2000, 100.

4. Bigazzi, Pierlugi, "Metals and Kidney Autoimmunity," *Environmental Health Perspectives,* 107 (supplement 5), Oct. 1999, 757.

5. Joint statement of the American Academy of Family Physicians, the American Academy of Pediatrics, the Advisory Committee on Immunization Practices, and the United States Public Health Service, July 14, 2000. Further information available at www.aafp.org/policy/camp/20.html.

6. Fox, Robert, MD, PhD, "Update on Systemic Lupus Erythematosus and Related Syndromes: Antiphospholipid Syndrome, Sjögren's Syndrome, and Myositis," *Medscape Conference Summaries from the American College of Rheumatology 2000 Annual Scientific Meeting,* Medscape, 2000, http://rheumatology.medscape.com/Medscape/CNO/2000/ACR/ACR-05.html.

7. Older, S., D. Battararno, et al., "Can Immunization Precipitate Connective Tissue Disease? Report of five cases of systemic lupus erythematosus and review of the literature," *Seminars in Arthritis and Rheumatology,* Dec. 1999; 29(3):131–139.

8. Hanchette, John, "Experts: Infant Vaccinations Linked to Autism, Conference urges testing of immune systems before shots are given," *The Denver Post,* via Gannett News Service, September 10, 2000, 20 A.

9. Bigazzi, Pierluigi, "Metals and Kidney Autoimmunity," *Environmental Health Perspectives* 107 (supplement 5) October 1999, 753–755.

10. Pollard, K. Michael, Deborah Pearson, et al., "Lupus-Prone Mice as Models to Study Xenobiotic-Induced Acceleration of Systemic Autoimmunity," *Environmental Health Perspectives* 107 (supplement 5) October 1999, 729–735.

11. Powell, Jonathan, Judy Van de Water, and M. Eric Gershwin, "Evidence for the Role of Environmental Agents in the Initiation or Progression of Autoimmune Conditions," *Environmental Health Perspectives* 107 (supplement 5) October 1999, 670.

12. Castranova, Vincent and Val Vallyathan, "Silicosis and Coal Worker's Pneumoconiosis," *Environmental Health Perspectives;* 108, supplement 4, August 2000, 675–684.

13. Kaufman, Mark, "Study Links Fibromyalgia, Ruptured Silicone Implants," *The Washington Post,* reprinted in the *Gazette Telegraph,* Colorado Springs, CO, May 1, 2001.

14. Shaheen, Victoria M., Minoru Satoh, Hanno B. Richards, et al., "Immunopathogenesis of Environmentally Induced Lupus in Mice," *Environmental Health Perspectives* 107, (supplement 5), October 1999, 723–727.

15. *Ibid.*

16. Freedman, D.M., Dosemeci, M., and M.C. Alavanja, "Mortality from Multiple Sclerosis and Exposure to Residential and Occupational Solar Radiation: A Case-Control Study Based on Death Certificates," *Occupational and Environmental Medicine,* June 2000, 57(6):418–421.

17. "Autoimmune Disease and the Environment," *Environmental Health Perspectives* 106(12), 1998, NIEH News via the internet, http://ehpnet1.niehs. nih.gov/docs/1998/106-12/niehsnews.html.

18. Smith, J. D., Terpening, C.M., et al., "Relief of Fibromyalgia Symptoms Following Discontinuation of Dietary Excitotoxins," *Annals of Pharmacotherapy,* June 2001, 35(6): 702–706.

19. Crinnion, Walter, ND, "Environmental Medicine, Part 4: Pesticides—Biologically Persistent and Ubiquitous Toxins," *Alternative Medicine Review,* 2000 Oct. 15(5):432–437.

20. "Pesticides and Aggression," *Rachel's Environment & Health Weekly,* # 648, April 29, 1999.

21. Holladay, Seven, "Prenatal Immunotoxicant Exposure and Postnatal Autoimmune Disease," *Environmental Health Perspectives* 107, supplement 5, Oct. 1999, 687–691.

22. Op. cit., Ravicz, 205.

23. Op. cit., Powell.

24. Wechsler, Pat, "A Shot in the Dark," *New York Magazine,* November 11, 1996, 39–44, 85.

25. Conlon, Paul, Jorge Oksenberg, et al., "The Immunobiology of Multiple Sclerosis: An autoimmune disease of the central nervous system," *Neurobiology of Disease;* 6: 146–149, 1999.

26. *Ibid.*

27. Altekruse, Sean, Norman Stern, et al., "Campylobacter jejuni: An Emerging Foodborne Pathogen," *Emerging Infectious Diseases;* 5(1), January-March 1999, via the CDC website, http://www.cdc.gov/ncidod/eid/vol5no1/ alterkruse.htm.

28. "Vaccine Victims? The Controversy Surrounding SmithKline Beecham's LYMErix," *ABC News,* New York, May 17, 2000, via the internet, http://abcnews.go.com/sections/living/ DailyNews/lyme_vaccine0516.html.

29. Yazbak, F. Edward, MD, FAAP, "Autism: Is There a Vaccine Connection? Part 1," *Vaccination after Delivery,* 1999; http://www.garynull.com/Documents/autism99b.htm.

30. "Study Supports Theory That Autism May Be Caused by an Immune System Response to a Virus," October 30, 1998, University of Michigan's College of Pharmacy/ *Medscape Wire* via the internet, http://www.medscape.com/MedscapeWire/1998/10.98/ medwire1030.autism.html.

31. "Parent Groups in US and Britain Charge Governments Manipulated Study Data to Stop Further Research into Vaccination and Autism," via the Vaccination Information Center website, the internet, http://www.909shot.com/wakefieldcriticism.htm.

32. Op. Cit., Hanchette.

33. "FDA Says There is No Link Between Most Vaccines, Autoimmune Diseases," *Reuters Ltd. Medical News*, Washington, D.C., May 4, 2000.

34. Stratton, Kathleen, et al., "DPT Vaccine and Chronic Nervous System Dysfunction: A New Analysis (1994)," *Congressional Quarterly Researcher*, August 25, 2000.

35. "Vaccine Injury Compensation: Program challenged to Settle Claims Quickly and Easily," Publication of the Government Accounting Office/Health and Human Services *GAO-00-8,* Letter Report 12/22/99.

36. Ovelgonne, J. H., J. Koninkx, et al., "Decreased Levels of Heat Shock Proteins in Gut Epithelial Cells after Exposure to Plant Lectins," *Gut,* 2000;46: 679.

37. Rao, Tharaknath and Bruce Richardson, "Environmentally Induced Autoimmune Diseases: Potential Mechanisms," *Environmental Health Perspectives*, Supplement 5, (107) October 5, 1999, 737–742.

38. Ramsaransing, G., Zwanikken, C., and J. De Keyser, "Worsening of Symptoms of Multiple Sclerosis Associated with Carbamazepine," Drugs Points in *British Medical Journal,* 2000, April 22; 320:1113.

39. Hess, Evelyn, "Are There Environmental Forms of Systemic Autoimmune Diseases?" *Environmental Health Perspectives* 107 (supplement 5) Oct 1999, 709–711.

40. Tremblay, Neil W. and Andrew P. Gilman, "Human Health, the Great Lakes, and Environmental Pollution: A 1994 Perspective," *Environmental Health Perspectives,* Supplement 9, December 1995, 103(9):3–5.

41. Klintschar, Michael, Patrizia Schwaiger, et al., "Evidence of Fetal Microchimerism in Hashimoto's Thyroiditis," *The Journal of Clinical Endocrinology & Metabolism;* 86(6):2494–2498.

42. Nelson, J. Lee, MD, "Microchimerism and Autoimmune Disease," Editorial in *New England Journal of Medicine,* April 23, 1998; 338(17): 1224–1225.

Chapter 6

1. Griggs, R., V. Askanas, et al., "Inclusion Body Myositis and Myopathies," *Annals of Neurology,* 1995; 38: 705–713.

2. Kavanaugh, Arther, MD, Russel Tomar, MD, John Reveille, MD, et al., Guidelines for Clinical Use of the "Antinuclear Antibody Test and Tests for Specific Autoantibodies to Nuclear Antigens," *in Archives of Pathology and Laboratory Medicine* 124:1–81, Chicago, College of American Pathologists, 2000.

3. *Ibid.*

4. *Ibid.*

5. Vernino, Steven, Phillip Low, et al., "Autoantibodies to Ganglionic Acetylcholine Receptors in Autoimmune Autonomic Neuropathies," *The New England Journal of Medicine,* Sept. 21, 2000, 343 (12): 847–855.

6. Peter, James, MD, PhD, *Use and Interpretation of Laboratory Tests in Neurology,* 4th Edition, Santa Monica, CA, Specialty Laboratories, 1994, 305.

7. Vernino, Steven, Phillip Low, et al., "Autoantibodies to Ganglionic Acetylcholine Receptors in Autoimmune Autonomic Neuropathies," *New England Journal of Medicine,* September 21, 2000; 343(12).

8. Leavelle, Dennis, MD, Editor, *Mayo Medical Laboratories Interpretive Handbook,* Rochester, MN, Mayo Medical Laboratories, 1997, 49.

9. Op. cit., Peter, 318.

10. *Ibid.,* 322.

11. *Ibid.,* 196.

12. *Ibid.*, 197.
13. Korula, Jacob, Liver Biopsy Role in the Management of Liver Disease, *Bombay Hospital Journal,* 38(4) October, 1996, Special Issue

Chapter 7

1. Petri, Michelle, MD, "Lupus in Men: Emotional and Physical Consequences," *In Focus,* Publication of the American Autoimmune and Related Diseases Association, Inc., Vol. 8(3), Sept. 2000.
2. Falk, Ronald, MD, "Treatment of Lupus Nephritis—A Work in Progress," *New England Journal of Medicine;* Oct. 19, 2000, 343(6):1182–1183.
3. Nakamura, Robert, MD, "Role of Autoantibody Tests in the Diagnostic Evaluation of Neuropsychiatric Systemic Lupus Erythematosus," in *Clinics in Laboratory Medicine,* Vol 17(3), September 1997, 379.
4. *Ibid.*, 381.
5. *Ibid.*
6. Centofani, Marjorie, "Salmonella's Molecular Mimics May Spark Arthritis, Study Shows," *The Gazette Online,* Johns Hopkins University, 29(21), Feb. 7, 2000.
7. Smith, Dorinda and Dori Germolec, "Introduction to Immunology and Autoimmunity," *Environmental Health Perspectives,* Vol. 107, supplement 5, Oct. 1999, 661–665.
8. House, Dorlinda, MD and William E. Winter, MD, "Autoimmune Diabetes, The Role of Autoantibody Markers in the Prediction and Prevention of Insulin Dependent Diabetes Mellitus," in *Clinics in Laboratory Medicine, Progress and Controversies in Autoimmune Disease Testing,* Philadelphia, W. B. Saunders, 1997, 499–545.
9. *Ibid.*
10. Classen, J. Barthelow, MD, "Vaccines Proven To Be Largest Cause of Insulin Dependent Diabetes in Children, Diabetics Advised to Seek Legal Counsel Now, Before Their Right to Compensation Expires," Classen Immunotherapies, Inc. website, http:www.vaccines.net/newage18.htm.
11. *Ibid.*
12. "Monoclonal Antibody Therapy for Crohn's Disease," publication of the Crohn's & Colitis Foundation of America via the internet, http:www.ccfa.org/medcentral/research/clinical/monoclon.htm.
13. "Autoimmunity," Natural Toxins Research Center at Texas A&M University, Kingsville, via the internet, http://ntri.tamuk.edu/immunology/autoimmunity.html.
14. Ward, B.J. PhD, McGill Center for Tropical Diseases, "Vaccine adverse events in the new millennium: Is there reason for concern," *Bulletin of the World Health Organization,* 2000, 78(20), 205–223.
15. Rosenfeld, Isadore, "When Your Nerves Can't 'Communicate'," *Parade Magazine,* May 20, 2001, 12.
16. Op. cit., Peter, 206–207.
17. *Ibid.*
18. Asa, Sylvia, MD, "The Dispersed Neuroendocrine Cell System," in *Functional Endocrine Pathology,* 2nd Edition, edited by Kalman Kovacs, MD, and Sylvia Asa, MD, Malden, MA, Blackwell Publishing, 1998, 1072.
19. Hellstrom, Wayne, MD, "Discoveries in Peyronie's Disease: Etiology, Prevalence, and Therapies," *Medscape* report from the American Urological Association 95th Annual Meeting, http:www.medscape.com/medscape/cno/2000/AUA.Sory.cfm?story_id=1323.
20. Schoen, Frederick, MD, Managing Editor, *Robbins Pathologic Basis of Disease,* 5th Edition, Philadelphia, W. B. Saunders, 1994, 370–371.
21. *Ibid.*, 493.

Chapter 8

1. Op. cit., Ravicz, 153.
2. Woodman, Richard, "Serious Blood Reactions Linked to Arthritis Drug," *Reuters Health*, London, October 10, 2000.
3. "Cancer Drug Approved for Treatment of MS," Associated Press release in *The Gazette Telegraph*, Colorado Springs, CO, October 14, 2000, A16.
4. Elkayam, O., Paran, D., et al., "Acute myocardial infarction associated with high dose intravenous immunoglobulin infusion for autoimmune disorders. A study of four cases," *Annals of Rheumatic Disease*, 2000, January; 59(1): 77–80.
5. Sherman, Neil, "New Drug Stalls Rheumatoid Arthritis, " *Health Scout*, January 4, 2001.
6. Berger, Abi, "Antibodies can repair damaged myelin in model of MS," *British Medical Journal*, News, June, 2000;320:1622.
7. Grando, Sergei, "Research Underway for the Development of Non-hormonal Treatment of Pemphigus," *In Focus*, Publication of AARDA, March, 2000; 8(1):7.
8. Antel, Jack, MD, "Neuroimmunology and Multiple Sclerosis Walking Tour," Highlights from the 124th Annual Meeting of the American Neurological Association, *Medscape*, 1999; http://www.medscape.com/Medscape/CNO/1999/ANA/ANA-01.html
9. "FDA Advisory Panel Recommends Approval of Drug for Treatment of Worsening Multiple Sclerosis," *In Focus*, Publication of AARDA, March, 2000; 8(1): 8–10.
10. Cockwell, P., Savage, C., et al. "Grand Rounds—Queen Elizabeth Medical Centre, Birmingham: Systemic Lupus Erythematosus, Complicated by Lupus, Nephritis and Antiphospholipid Antibody Syndrome," *British Medical Journal*, January 1997, 314: 292.
11. Op. cit., Fox.
12. *Ibid.*

Chapter 9

1. Op cit., Ravicz, 110.
2. Hart, Marybeth, "Study Suggests Tart Cherries May Ease Arthritis," *The Gazette Telegraph*, May 16, 2001, Life5.
3. McCarty, M.F., "Upregulation of Lymphocyte Apoptosis as a Strategy for Preventing and Treating Autoimmune Disorders: A Role for Whole-Food Vegan Diets, Fish Oil and Dopamine Agonists," *Medical Hypotheses*, 2001, July; 57(2):258–275.
4. Op. cit., Ravicz, 32.
5. Ross, Catherine, "New Light Shed on Vitamin A's Role in the Body's Natural Defenses," April 2, 2001, *Penn State Newsletter*.
6. Op. Cit., Ravicz, 178.
7. *Ibid.*, 267.
8. Mowatt, Twig, "Lose the Fear, Stronger than she ever imagined—despite MS," *Life Extension*, April, 2000; 6(4): 57–59.
9. Twombly, Renee, "Painfully Icy Fingers Could Mean Raynaud's" *OnHealth*, November 23, 1998, via the internet, http://onhealth.webmd.com/conditions/in-depth/item/itempercentC33823_1_1.asp.
10. Op. cit., Ravicz, 242.
11. *Ibid.*, 162.
12. Borysenko, Joan, *The Power of the Mind to Heal, Renewing Body, Mind and Spirit*, Audio Series, Niles, IL, Nightingale Conant, 1993, (800) 323–5552.
13. "Can Stress Make You Sick?" *Harvard Health Letter*, April, 1998; 23(6); 1–2.
14. Gottlieb, Scott, "Cannabinoids Might Reduce Spasticity in Multiple Sclerosis," *British Medical Journal* News Section, 2000, March 320:666.

Chapter 10

1. Krimsky, Sheldon, *Hormonal Chaos, The Scientific and Social Origins of the Environmental Endocrine Hypothesis,* Baltimore, Johns Hopkins Press, 2000, 228–230.

2. Fagin, Dan and Marianne Lavelle and the Center for Public Integrity, *Toxic Deception: How the Chemical Industry Manipulates Science, Bends the Law and Endangers Your Health,* Monroe, Maine, Common Courage Press, 1999, x.

3. Op. cit., Krimsy, 124–125.

4. Pieters, Raymond and Ruud Albers, "Screening Tests for Autoimmune-related Immunotoxicity," *Environmental Health Perspectives,* Supplement 5, (107) October 5, 1999, 673–678.

5. Ferriman, Annabel, "Attempts to ban DDT have had 'tragic consequences,'" *British Medical Journal,* News roundup, May 2001; 322:1270.

6. Bernard, Sallie and Lyn Redwood, "On Slowing Quicksilver to a Stop," *Feat Daily Newsletter,* Sacramento, California, Dec. 1, 2000.

7. Backous, Douglas, "Autoimmune Inner Ear Disease," Publication of the Bobby R. Alford Department of Otorhinolaryngology and Communicative Sciences, April 1993.

8. Ji-Won Yoon, Chang-Soon Yoon, Hye-Won Lim, et al., *"Control of Autoimmune Diabetes in NOD Mice by GAD Expression or Suppression* in ß Cells," Science 1999; 284:1183–1187.

9. "Possible New Treatment for IBD Suggested," *In Focus,* Publication of AARDA, March 2000; 8(1):8.

10. Rose, Noel, "The Autoimmune Diseases," *In Focus,* Publication of AARDA, June 2001; 9(2): 6.

11. Op. Cit., Conlon.

12. *Ibid.*

13. *Ibid.*

14. Traynor, A.E., et al., "Treatment of severe systemic lupus erythematosus with high-dose chemotherapy and haematopoietic stem-cell transplantation: A phase E study," *Lancet,* 2000, 356:701.

15. "Stem Cell Research Paves the Way for a Potential Cure for Type 1 Diabetes," *Reuters Medical News* at Medscape via the internet, August 15, 2000.

16. Lynden, Patricia, "Scorpion Venom Halts Autoimmune Diseases, Chemical in poison suppresses immune system," *Health Scout Reporter,* July 11, 2000.

17. Davis, Thomas, "Monoclonal Antibodies for Hematologic Malignancies: Current Options, Future Directions," *Oncology Treatment Updates,* Medscape, 2000

Index